HIDDEN DEPTHS

For Mary

Best wishes

Sue Hennessy

4 March 2016

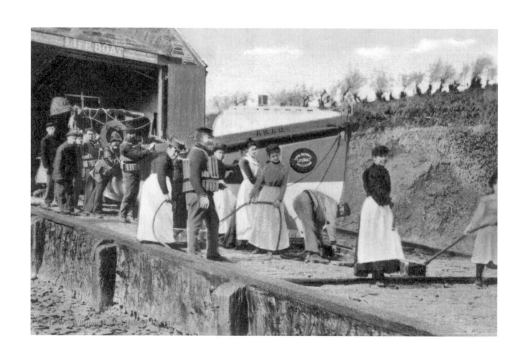

HIDDEN DEPTHS

DEPTHS

Women of the RNLI

SUE HENNESSY

The History Press

For Alan
Always my great encourager and who, like me,
so admired the women of the RNLI

Frontispiece Page 2: Launching the lifeboat, Padstow. (Iain Booth postcard collection)
Page 6: 'The Call to Duty'. (Iain Booth postcard collection)

First published 2010

The History Press
The Mill, Brimscombe Port
Stroud, Gloucestershire, GL5 2QG
www.thehistorypress.co.uk

British Library Cataloguing in Publication Data.
A catalogue record for this book is available from the British Library.

ISBN 978 0 7524 5443 6

Typesetting and origination by The History Press
Printed in Great Britain
Manufacturing managed by Jellyfish Print Solutions Ltd

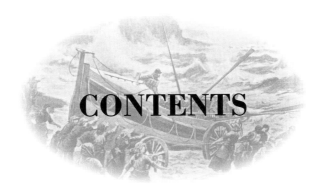

CONTENTS

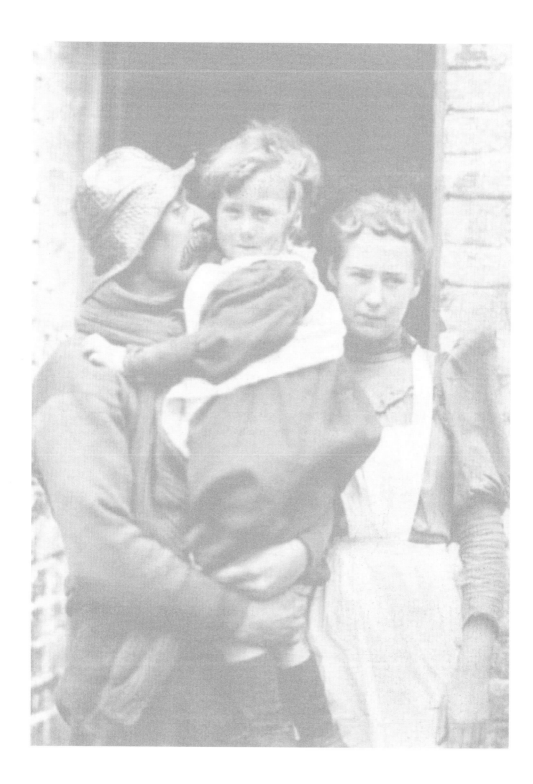

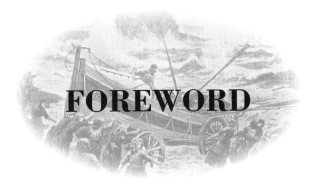

FOREWORD

Sometimes the wives and partners of the Royal National Lifeboat Institution crew are forgotten as the great British public continues its admiration of the amazing and courageous work carried out by the UK's lifeboat men. But those women have always been – and fiercely remain – the loyal and hardworking champions of their crew, in every sense. They not only accept but actively encourage and take pride in every member of the boat as he or she embarks on each often dangerous mission. Nor does this support belong to the past: each generation maintains a similar respect and acknowledgement not only of the task of the lifeboat crew, but also the high esteem in which they are held nationwide.

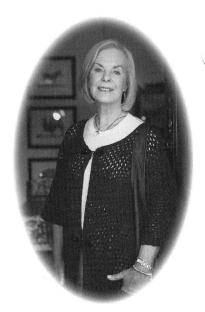

Her Royal Highness, The Duchess of Kent

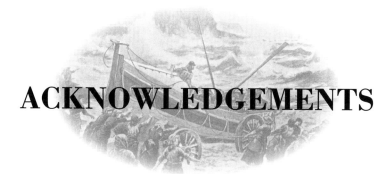

ACKNOWLEDGEMENTS

The idea of writing a book to document and celebrate the achievements of the women of the RNLI has long been in my mind. I carried the thought with me throughout my working years, knowing that I would need the time and space afforded by retirement to make it happen. It is my first major project since completing my career with the RNLI.

The many people who have helped me have also made the journey a very special experience and I hope that, as well as accepting my thanks, they will share my pleasure in what we have created.

My special thanks go to Ray and Susannah Kipling who, as experienced book authors, helped point me in the right direction and gave encouragement at the right time. As did Brian Miles, who shared his vivid memories of the many RNLI women he has met over the years.

At the RNLI, I have been given great help and advice by Barry Cox and Peter Moorman, Michael Vlasto, Brian Wead, Joanna Bellis, Carolyn Anand, Sarah Sleigh, Sue Fernley, Alison Sheward and Caroline Smith. Derek King, before leaving, patiently took me through the image library. Rory Stamp has given great help since then. Liz Cook coordinated the contact I needed within the organisation and was a good guide on 'matters writing'. For their great help and endless patience, warmest thanks go to my editors, Emily Locke and Amy Rigg.

The willing and enthusiastic help of so many RNLI friends around the coast was vital. I thank you all, but must mention Richard Martin, Frank Kilroy, David Forshaw and Iain Booth in particular.

Having friends who will tell you the absolute truth when you say to them 'read that – what do you think?' is a wonderful asset and I was blessed with Doreen Hinchliffe, Cherry Hambrook and Rachel Blake. My thanks to you all are boundless.

Very importantly though, my warmest thanks go to the very many women who agreed to be involved – you have confirmed my absolute belief in the power of women to make good, and sometimes quite exceptional, things happen.

Sadly, three people who feature in this book died while it was being written: Patricia Kellehar, Evelyn Paley and Richard Davies.

Author note: Images without a source were donated for inclusion within the book with no request for a credit.

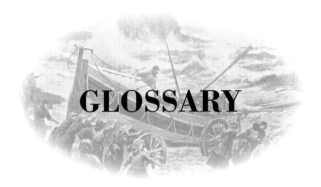

GLOSSARY

ALB   *All-weather lifeboat* – Lifeboats designed and built to withstand hurricane conditions and to selfright from complete capsize.

ILB   *Inshore Lifeboat* – Lifeboats designed and built with the capability of operating close to the shore in shallow water. Open to the elements, they can be righted by the crew after capsize.

Coxswain   The person in command of an ALB and who has complete responsibility for the lifeboat and the crew while afloat.

Helm   The person driving an ALB or ILB, and the person in command of an ILB.

Mechanic   Member of the crew who has responsibility for the day-to-day (first line) maintenance of the lifeboat, such that it is always in a fit state to go to sea. At an all-weather station, the coxswain is sometimes also the mechanic.

SHS   *Station Honorary Secretary* (replaced in 2003 by LOM, see below) – Leading voluntary role at each lifeboat station with responsibilities that include authorising the launch of a lifeboat, providing RNLI HQ with a record of each lifeboat service, administration of crew information.

LOM   *Lifeboat Operations Manager* – Who, as a volunteer, has all the same responsibilities of the SHS role plus others, including local maintenance of the lifeboat station, management of all volunteers and public relations.

DLA   *Deputy Launching Authority* – A local volunteer who, in the absence of the LOM, is authorised to give permission for the lifeboat to launch.

Shore Helper   One of a team of volunteers who enable the launch and recovery of a lifeboat.

Lifeboat
Inspector   A staff member with responsibility in the division for operational staff and volunteers, the station premises, lifeboats and other equipment, as well as training and assessment.

MCA   *Maritime and Coastguard Agency* – The agency of the UK Government that includes HM Coastguard, responsible for the initiation and coordination of all civilian maritime Search and Rescue (SAR) activity.

'Shout'   The informal term for a lifeboat call out on service.

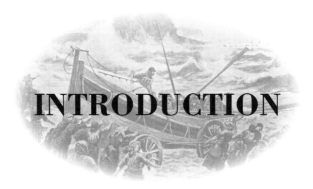

INTRODUCTION

When we hear the word 'lifeboats' or 'RNLI', the first picture to jump into our minds will almost certainly be that of a big, brave, bearded lifeboat man. With good reason, as for over 180 years such images of strong, selfless males have populated many of the reports and literature of the lifeboat service. What has not been so well documented or recognised are the roles that, right from the very beginning, women have played in working to save lives at sea. Perhaps the stereotypical image is of women waiting in the lifeboat station for their men to return – brewing tea and giving solace and encouragement to one another.

Look more deeply, though, and it is clear that women have always been at the heart of the RNLI operation, undertaking a wide range of tasks which draw upon their distinctive skills and talents. Their contribution continues to expand as the organisation itself grows and develops. Look at the women of the RNLI in the twenty-first century and we find them involved in virtually every activity and at every level of responsibility. Given that most women do not naturally seek recognition for themselves, much of the female history of the lifeboat service has never been captured. Even so, it would take a book far bigger than this to give a comprehensive account of all the many thousands of women who, in one way or another, have served the RNLI – so significant is the part they have played.

The women featured in this book have volunteered to participate knowing that they are representatives for all those others who have made and continue to make similar contributions. The author is very keen to receive further stories and information about 'women of the RNLI' – please send them to her via the publishers.

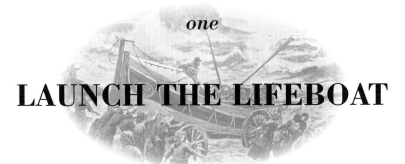

one

LAUNCH THE LIFEBOAT

Think of a lifeboat rescue. What are the images that immediately come to mind? You will probably picture a very hostile environment; there are raging seas, howling gales and bone chilling cold. On the sea there is a lifeboat making its perilous way to the casualty where there are people in danger of drowning. Most people will see the lifeboat crew – strong, brave men, risking their own lives to go to the rescue of others.

What is unlikely to feature in your imagining is how the lifeboat got there or how it was launched into the sea. There is not a lot of glamour in launching and recovering lifeboats – but it has to be done. This much less conspicuous element of a lifeboat rescue is both physically demanding and dangerous. Who did it in the early days of the lifeboat service? You may be surprised to learn that the answer is women.

It was they who heaved heavy lifeboats down the beach, pulled on harsh ropes, struggled with the ups and downs of the uneven beach, waded into the sea – sometimes out of their depth – unleashed the lifeboat in the swirling water and hurried to get clear before being hit. Most probably they would have been coping with wild weather, darkness, the wind and the rain tearing into them and the sea spray would clog their eyes with salt, painfully exposing every little cut and abrasion on hands and legs. For them, there was no scientifically engineered personal protection equipment to wear, just their everyday clothes which were completely inadequate. A headscarf might give a little protection but just imagine how those cold, waterlogged skirts would cling to their freezing bodies.

Initially, it was the men in a coastal community who volunteered to crew the lifeboats. They combined this commitment with earning their living, most usually as fishermen or some other occupation related to the sea. It was a hard life and they worked long hours. Their wives would have worked hard too, but this was usually within the family home or within the village. The men would not have wanted their wives to help with crewing the lifeboat, as there were deeply held views that women would bring them danger at sea. But women could – and did – play a part in helping their men in the lifeboat service, and their contribution was an essential one.

Along all parts of the coastline, women supported their men on the lifeboat crews by working together to get the lifeboat afloat and then later recovering it from the water in readiness for when the next call came. Without question, theirs is a major contribution to the cause of saving life at sea and one which has often been eclipsed by the relative excitement of what actually happened at sea. Much of their work went unrecorded, but from what has been documented in north-east England, and also at Dungeness on the south coast, it is possible to begin to understand what magnificent feats of strength and teamwork these courageous and dedicated women launchers performed.

Northumberland

Cresswell

Cresswell is a small village on the coast of Northumberland, just twenty miles north of the River Tyne. For many years it was a fishing village with the distinction that a high percentage of the residents were named Brown – people who from time immemorial were renowned for their giant stature and hardiness.

Margaret Brown was born the daughter of a fisherman. At thirteen she left school to help her father and brothers with the female tasks associated with fishing: digging for bait, mending nets, making crab pots and hauling up the cobles – locally built fishing boats – onto the beach. Her settled life changed dramatically in 1874, when a sudden summer storm claimed the lives of her father and three of her brothers as their coble was caught by a huge breaker. Margaret was on the beach with friends and neighbours, desperately hoping for their safe landing. Instead she had the heartbreaking task of pulling their bodies out of the sea.

A positive outcome from this tragedy was that the RNLI placed a lifeboat at Cresswell that same year. Margaret made the decision to involve herself fully with the lifeboat service and immediately helped with the launching and recovery work. She went on to live until 1928 and in all that time never missed a launch. There is evidence she helped with many difficult rescues and experienced the harshness of wild conditions on numerous occasions, but one 'shout' stands out, and it took place just two years after Cresswell Lifeboat Station was established.

In the early hours of January 1876 in a gale and torrential rain, the German ship *Gustaf* got into serious trouble off Druridge Bay. Such were the conditions that it was difficult to launch the lifeboat and it had to be dragged for half a mile along soft sand until a suitable place was found. By now the situation for those on board the *Gustaf* was desperate; the ship had struck rocks and, worse still, there were men in the water. The Cresswell women formed a human chain to try to reach them – Margaret was at the extreme end of it and completely out of her depth, and other women were being swept off their feet by the waves. The coxswain made courageous attempts to reach the wreck but to no avail, realising that they needed to get the Rocket Life-Saving Apparatus from Newbiggin, about five miles away.

Three women volunteered to go: Margaret Brown, Isabella Armstrong and Mary Brown. The coxswain put Margaret in charge even though he could see she was already exhausted. What followed was a desperate run by the young women down the coast, across swollen rivers and bleak moorland. So great was the wind that they decided to scramble down the cliffs and proceed along the beach, but then they nearly got washed away by the huge

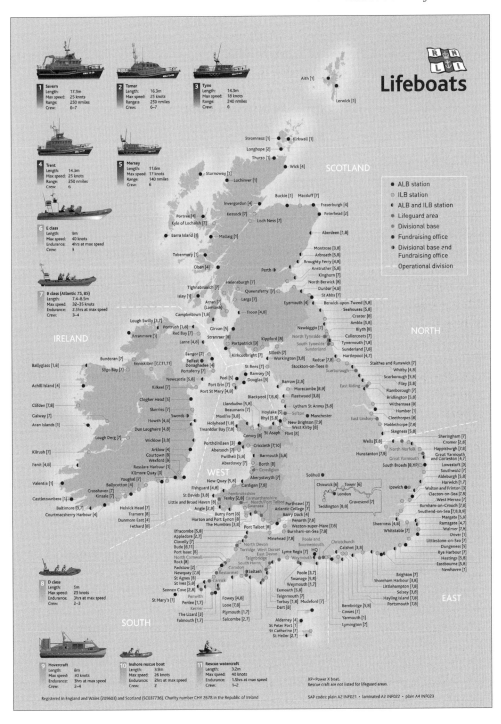

RNLI rescue map 2010.

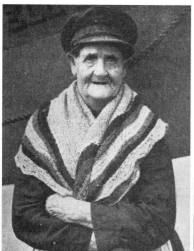

Left Margaret Armstrong (formerly Brown) of Cresswell in 1922 – she never missed a launch in fifty years. (Central Press)

Below Launching the lifeboat at Cresswell in 1927. (Topical Press Agency)

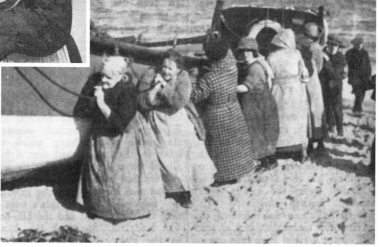

waves. On the outskirts of Newbiggin, Isabella and Mary dropped to the ground with exhaustion and, having found a cottage to take them in, Margaret ran on alone. Eventually she reached Newbiggin coastguard station and collapsed, unable even to speak. Fortunately she was well known in those parts and the coastguard was able to work out what was wrong and send the Apparatus by horses straight away.

The result was a happy one. All ten people on the *Gustaf* were saved – but, ironically, after all that effort, not by the Apparatus. In fact, the lifeboat had made a second successful rescue attempt before it arrived. The courage and endurance of the three young women was recognised by both the coastguard and the RNLI. In spite of her harrowing experience that night, Margaret was clearly motivated to continue launching the lifeboat and in 1922, by now Mrs Margaret Armstrong, she was awarded the Gold Brooch by the RNLI in recognition of her long service.

The description of her funeral in 1928, written by the District Organising Secretary for the North of England, Edgar Johnson, confirms the respect and admiration that Margaret commanded within the RNLI both locally and nationally:

As Margaret Armstrong was reverently borne outside her cottage a large gathering sang the fishermen's hymn. Then lifted on the shoulders of four stalwart life-boatmen, she was taken up the hill to the little Parish Church, the only wreath on her coffin being that sent by the Institution in the form of an anchor, with the words, 'The Royal National Life-boat Institution's last mark of respect' ... a congregation of over 200 from miles around filled the little place of worship ... we deplored her passing but rejoiced in the thought that we had had the privilege in knowing her. She had gone to her last home a shining example to the women of the British Isles.

While the story of Margaret is very special, two other women from Cresswell, both wives of coxswains, are notable for the great support they gave. Kitty, wife of William Brown, was a launcher for fifty years and actually performed a single-handed rescue of three fishermen by launching a small boat and rowing to them. As well as answering the telephone at the lifeboat station, she did much to raise funds. The wife of James Brown, second coxswain, also gave fifty years' service as a launcher.

Newbiggin

A dramatic headline in *London Illustrated* in 1941 declared 'Newbiggin breeds Britain's toughest women', and it could very well be correct, for the record of achievement over many years by the female launchers from its community is remarkable. It is with transparent pride that the female launchers of Newbiggin are referred to as 'Our Women', and although there are no women launching lifeboats there today, the term lives on as their fervent support continues in other ways.

Like Cresswell, Newbiggin had its beginnings as a small fishing community and there has been a lifeboat stationed there since 1851. Rarely were horses used to launch the lifeboat and women took a major responsibility for launching. In fact the shout 'Every man to the boat, every woman to the rope' was frequently heard when the lifeboat was needed. This they have done on hundreds of occasions, but there were two exceptional launches for which the women of Newbiggin were officially recognised by the RNLI with Thanks on Vellum in 1927 and 1940.

On an apparently fine day in January 1927 the whole of the Newbiggin fishing fleet went out but was caught in an unexpected gale. The coxswain had a problem as the crew was already at sea. Fortunately, he had the wives to launch the lifeboat. Aboard was an inexperienced crew he had anxiously pulled together. The women had an extremely difficult time in very adverse conditions and although the official RNLI record tells the story well, it is the first-hand account of one of the launchers, Bella Arkle, given in an interview with the *Evening Chronicle* fifty-three years later, which really paints the picture:

Rain speared down from black skies, a howling freezing gale tore at the roots of the fishermen's cottages by the shoreline, a boiling sea was thundering ashore with huge combers breaking over the rocks in a fury of spume. Out there tossing and corkscrewing among the huge waves lay the entire fishing fleet of Newbiggin, among them almost the entire lifeboat crew. Today was to be the day the women of Newbiggin, the fishermen's wives, saved their men folk. It was always the tradition for the women to launch the lifeboat – you had to go into the water up to your neck to get the boat out. By 11a.m. there was no indication that the weather would ease with wind at gale force and, it was freezing and raining. The lifeboat would

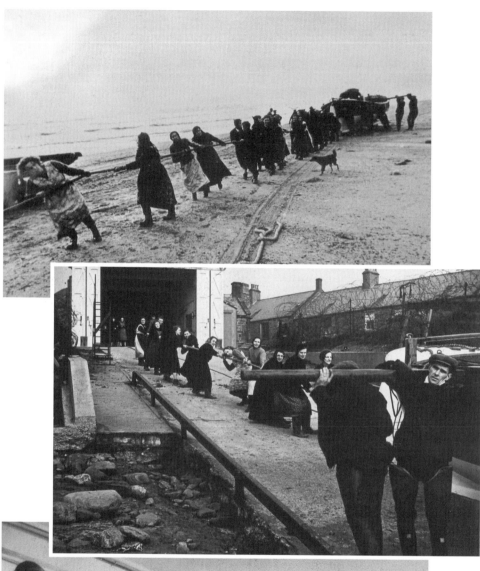

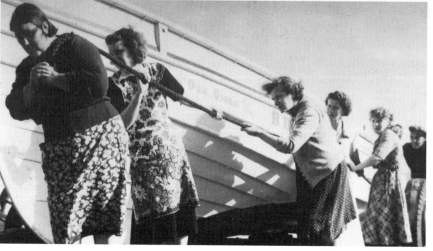

Right and opposite Launching the lifeboat at Newbiggin. (Newbiggin Heritage Partnership)

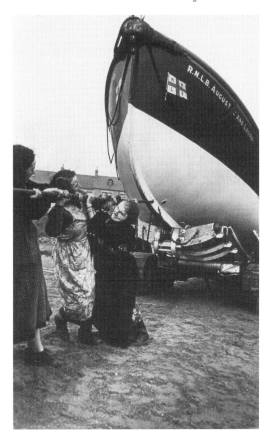

have to be launched with a scratch crew and one was forthcoming, it needed only a phone call to the colliery manager. Along came a crew of pitmen with muck still in their faces. I was working as a cleaner said Bella, and when the alarm went off I ran to the lifeboat house where all the women were gathering. The weather had really turned bad when the lifeboat was brought out and got into the water but waves threw it back. We had to straighten her up by wading right in. I was up to my neck that day, but we managed to get the boat away and all the fishing boats were brought back safely. In fact the boat was out for three hours and the Newbiggin womenfolk for the most part waited on the foreshore in their wet clothes, facing into the gale, to help haul the lifeboat in. That too was the tradition.

An account of their role in the rescues, along with that of the black-faced miners, was broadcast by the BBC, and responses were received from all over the country.

'Our women' had many more soakings between 1926 and 1940, but with their usual modesty and steadfastness they just got on with it. One of the station's most difficult launches in February 1940 would bring recognition for their determination and courage a second time. The launch was to go to the rescue of a vessel that had gone aground in stormy weather. In the darkness of an early morning in winter the women rose from their beds and assisted with the launch, only to discover that the lifeboat had a failing engine which prevented it from making way – in fact a huge wave drove it back onto the beach. A decision was made to take the lifeboat overland, which meant across some rough terrain, so that it could be launched nearer to the stranded ship.

More helpers were summoned and eventually sixty people – many of them women – gathered to haul the lifeboat overland across the undulating moors and over rocky ground to a place where it could be launched. After the monumental effort, the launchers waited and watched while eleven people were rescued from the ship and taken away in an ambulance. The job was far from over, though. Now the lifeboat had to be recovered from the sea, hauled up the beach and back across the moors to Newbiggin. After much effort the lifeboat arrived back at its station at 11a.m. This was a rescue that had started at 4.50a.m. The second Thanks on Vellum presented by the RNLI to the women launchers was very well deserved.

Eventually, in 1949, Newbiggin took delivery of a tractor which would from then on do the work of launching the lifeboat – a wonderful development for all those women who froze in the sea, got innumerable cuts and bruises, and ruined many of their clothes. Free from their launching duties 'Our Women' still wanted to be an integral part of saving lives at sea in their community, and thus turned their energies and enthusiasm to fundraising. Predictably, they did this very well!

Holy Island

Twenty-five women received a Letter of Thanks from the RNLI in recognition of their 'fine spirit of humane and helpful service' when they assisted with a desperately difficult launch in January 1922 which required the labours of sixty people to execute. In the dark and blinding snow they hauled the lifeboat across deep mud and waded waist deep in the sea so that the lifeboat could reach a suitable launching point to go to a stranded ship. After launching, the rescue required daring seamanship to save the lives of nine men, for which the RNLI awarded the coxswain a Silver Medal. Fulsome praise for the women was given in the *Berwick Journal*, which described them as 'Grace Darlings – every one'.

Boulmer

Boulmer was a small village with just thirty-four houses in the 1920s, yet there were thirty-five women on the launching team. Boulmer women received Thanks on Vellum awards from the RNLI twice. The first was for their great efforts to help the Craster fishermen on 24 March 1924 when they were unable to make the harbour because of the heavy seas. Boulmer men were out fishing too, so an ex-coxswain took charge. This was going to be a difficult launch at low tide and, having been mustered, all the women of Boulmer were soon up to their knees in mud and then up to their waists in water. It was a great struggle and two of the women were overcome by cold and exhaustion and had to be carried home, but the lifeboat was eventually under way and helped some of the fishermen to safety.

A year later on 20 December 1925, the women were roused from their beds at 3a.m. to launch the lifeboat in a blizzard to go to a ship that had gone aground on rocks. They had to haul the heavy boat over difficult terrain, but their perseverance meant the lifeboat was eventually launched into heavy seas at 7a.m. Try as he might, though, the coxswain could not reach the casualty, and with the tide rapidly going out, the lifeboat was recovered by the waiting women. Desperate to help the men stranded on the ship, they then heaved it along a lane so narrow that the wheels kept sinking in the ditches and the horse that was helping decided to stop and go no further. The women battled on to a place further along the coast to try to reach a better launching site. Alnmouth lifeboat had by now launched and so the Boulmer lifeboat was no longer needed, but the launchers stood by for another two hours – just in case! On that wild night, they had been on duty for almost seven hours.

Two of the women – Miss N. Stephenson, daughter of the coxswain, and Mrs B. Stanton, wife of the second coxswain – went to London to receive the second award. It must have been immensely exciting because neither had been further south than the Tyne before. To help them feel comfortable, the Duke of Northumberland invited them to stay at his London home. Before the ceremony they went to lay a wreath at the Cenotaph, in memory of the Boulmer men who had lost their lives in the First World War.

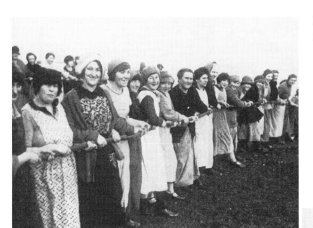

Launching the lifeboat at Boulmer, 1926. (R. Bell Bolton – Amble)

Launching the lifeboat at Boulmer, 1925. (Iain Booth postcard collection)

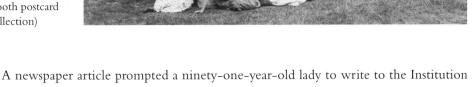

A newspaper article prompted a ninety-one-year-old lady to write to the Institution enclosing a donation:

> I read with the greatest interest the account in the *Morning Post* of the thirty-five women at Boulmer who got out the Life-boat on a December night, and that you are going to express your appreciation of their bravery. I am a Northumbrian woman, born two years before our beloved Queen Victoria came to the throne. I lived there for nearly forty years, and still keep the memory of the good brave women I knew in those days, and am so glad there are still some like them.
>
> I remember seeing the Life-boats and rockets in use at Tynemouth before the North and South Piers were built, and once, unhappily, saw a vessel with all on board lost in one of the rough NE seas – so you will understand why I always read about Northumberland and the Life-boats. I have seen Bamburgh and Grace Darling's home, and Alnwick, that of the Duchess of Northumberland, who is taking an interest also in this case.
>
> I wish I could send you a donation for each of the thirty-five, but reduced income and other claims prevent this, but the enclosed will just show that, although far away, my dear old county is still remembered. If you have an opportunity to privately tell your two visitors how I have thought of them I will be glad. Wishing your Society great success.

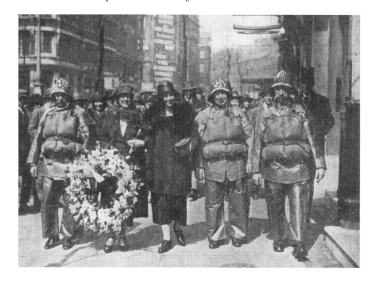

Miss Stephenson and Mrs Stanton from Boulmer with Coxwains Cross (Humber), Fleming (Gorleston) and Dobson (Donna Nook) in 1926, on their way to lay a wreath at the Cenotaph in memory of the men of Boulmer who died in the First World War. (Central Press)

PS. – You can either let the money help to entertain them here or go to the funds of the Society as you think best. Excuse my shaky writing.

Just how strong these women were is exemplified by Mrs Stephenson who, as both a daughter and wife of a Boulmer coxswain, had always been involved in launching the lifeboat and thought nothing of going into the water on a bitter winter day. It is recorded that in 1921, when she was already sixty-three years old, she struggled for two hours up to her waist in the sea to get the boat afloat. When this particular rescue took place she had only a couple more years to live. She must have had many fearful experiences, but said that her worst was when both her father and husband had to stay in the lifeboat riding at anchor all night. The launching carriage had been washed away and because the wind and tide were so strong, the lifeboat could not return to shore. Next morning Mrs Stephenson saw only a piece of the carriage sticking out of the sea and immediately thought that the lifeboat and crew were lost. Happily this was not so – the lifeboat had moved in the night.

Tyne and Wear

Cullercoats

At Cullercoats, a few miles further south on the North Sea coast, the women were just as used to turning out in all weathers to launch the lifeboat and did not hesitate when the call came soon after daybreak on 1 January 1861. A ship – *Lovely Nelly* – had been seen flying a distress flag and the lifeboat was urgently needed. The weather could not have been worse, with high winds and driving snow. The sea was raging as, with great determination, the lifeboat was dragged for two miles through the gale by Cullercoats villagers, many of them women, and then launched close to Brier Dene. The crew rowed across the heavy seas and skilfully placed their lifeboat alongside the *Lovely Nelly.* With no time to spare, the six men crawled into the safety of the lifeboat.; all, that is, but one – the twelve-year-old cabin boy

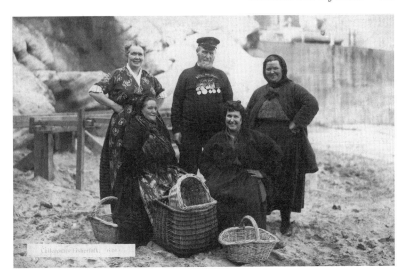

Cullercoats
fisherwomen
with Coxswain
Robert Smith
of Tynemouth
(Polly Donkin
far right). (Iain
Booth postcard
collection)

who was too afraid to jump from the rigging and, in spite of all the efforts to save him, fell into the sea and drowned.

This dramatic launch was depicted in a painting, 'The Women', by John Charlton, which now hangs in the Laing Gallery, Newcastle. Painted several years later in 1910, it shows the Cullercoats women taking a major role in hauling the lifeboat. To be strictly accurate, it should have shown the horses which helped with the arduous task, but that does not diminish the magnificent achievements of the women and men who launched the lifeboat on that dreadful New Year's Day.

This was confirmed by all who took part in a reconstruction of the event in 2008. Organised for the BBC series *Coast*, volunteers, including members of the current Cullercoats crew, pulled the lifeboat along the same route that had been taken in 1861. It was a huge challenge, which gave all who took part and those who watched some insight into what the lifeboat launchers in years gone by had endured. Robert Oliver, a helmsman on Cullercoats crew who follows five generations involved with the lifeboat, said after he had completed the pull: 'I believe they should have had medals the size of frying pans.'

Cleveland

Redcar

A launch at Redcar in 1921 ended very tragically with the accidental loss of a young woman's life. A number of Redcar fishing cobles had bravely gone to the aid of a colliery ship that had gone aground. They tried to help the ship get clear of the rocks, but as the weather worsened they had to return to shore. There they discovered that six Redcar men had been left behind. They and the crew of the *Aphrodite* were in danger so, in a terrific gale, preparations were made to launch the lifeboat.

Many bystanders helped and, following the great tradition of women helping to launch the lifeboat, women grabbed the ropes too. In the great effort, one woman stumbled and

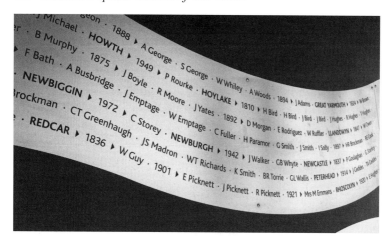

The only woman named on the RNLI Memorial sculpture – Margaret Emmans from Redcar. (RNLI/Rory Stamp)

brought down several others. This was when tragedy struck. A young woman who had only recently been married fell into the path of the lifeboat and was crushed to death. So recent was her wedding that she was known to many as Margaret Crosby, but she was actually Margaret Emmans when she died. Little more is known about her, but she is the only woman to appear on the RNLI Memorial to those who lost their lives in the attempt to save others at sea.

Yorkshire

Runswick

When the fishermen of Runswick, who happened to be the lifeboat crew, were caught in an unexpected storm on 12 April 1901, their wives launched the lifeboat while a scratch crew was found to go to their rescue. The women had to wade into the water to get the lifeboat off and then, soaking wet, wait for almost three hours on the beach until every man was safely landed.

North Devon

Lynmouth

While much of the evidence for the role played by women in launching lifeboats has been preserved in the north of England, there is no doubt that women from all around our coast were involved in this demanding and dangerous work. Like so much of what was done by men at lifeboat stations to save lives, the part played by women launchers was taken for granted and, as such, was overlooked.

The story of the remarkable launch of the Lynmouth lifeboat on 12 January 1899 is one of the better known pieces of RNLI history. A large ship was in distress in the Bristol Channel but conditions were too bad to launch the lifeboat at Lynmouth. The agreed solution was to launch from Porlock. The road from Lynmouth to Porlock, of great notoriety

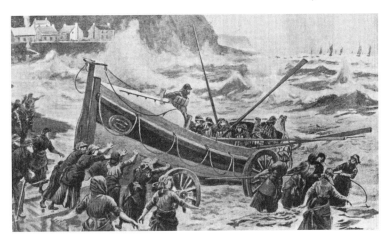

Runswick women launching the lifeboat.

even today, has two of the steepest hills in England: Countisbury and Porlock. At one point it ascends 1500ft in two miles. Every available man and woman set out – there were twenty-eight in all. With a gale blowing, in driving rain and in the pitch dark, they hauled the heavy wooden lifeboat though lanes and across fields, having sometimes to remove farm gates and posts. At one point a wheel came off and had to be replaced, and at another the road had washed away. It took ten and a half hours to reach Porlock, which they did without casualty. Then they waited until the following morning before joining two tugs which took the ship *Forrest Hall* to Barry. Here thankfully the lifeboat crew were given food, as they had not eaten for twenty-four hours. The group of launchers had made their weary way back to Lynmouth on foot. Soaking wet, they too had not eaten since setting out the previous night.

The story may have ended differently if one woman who they met on the way had put a spanner in the works. She lived in a cottage at the bottom of Porlock Hill and had been woken by the sound of part of her cottage being demolished by the launchers to make way for the lifeboat to get through. Angrily, she demanded to know what right they had 'bringing a thing like that at this time of night, knocking down people's walls and waking them up'. She was much surprised to learn that it was a lifeboat as she had never seen one before. On being told about the ship in distress and of their endeavours to rescue the men, she decided to join them for the rest of the journey.

Kent

Dungeness

Dungeness was a top security area during the Second World War, but the work of the lifeboat continued. Minefields on either side of the slipway created additional dangers for the launchers, leaving only a narrow space where they could stand. The doodlebugs were another hazard if a shout came when they were about.

In 1979, Dungeness Lifeboat Station received a tractor and its arrival signalled the end of many years of manual lifeboat launching across what is a very bleak and challenging shingle

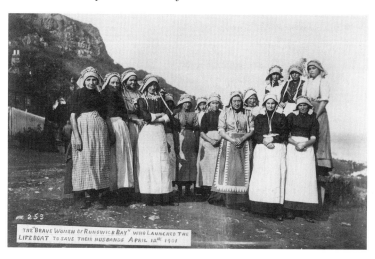

Postcard of Runswick women launchers involved in the 1901 rescue of their own husbands. (Iain Booth postcard collection)

headland, with no protective harbour and no sea defences. Dungeness is a remote place steeped in history, and it is not really surprising that the traditional methods of lifeboat launching saw out their last days here.

The launch is particularly difficult; the start from the boathouse is down a slipway, but at its end the remainder of the shore has to be made over heavy wooden skids. Positioning these in the pathway of the lifeboat requires both strength and skill, and it has to be right or else there is risk to the boat and the human beings working around it. The wind can easily deflect the course of the lifeboat and so great judgement is needed to compensate for this. If things go wrong, it may be necessary to start all over again. As with other stations, the launchers almost always had to wade into the sea.

Such was the challenge that the women launchers of Dungeness were held in high esteem and with real justification. They have twice been awarded Thanks on Vellum by the RNLI. First in 1932, when it took thirty-seven launchers, fourteen of whom were women, to launch the lifeboat in a gale and very heavy rain. The aim was to go to the rescue of a London barge – the *Shamrock* – in trouble with three men aboard. So strong was the wind that on the first attempt a sudden gust blew the lifeboat right off the skids and on to the beach. With huge effort it had to be hauled up again to replace the skids. The launchers were by now soaked to the skin and had difficulty keeping a footing on the shingle, but they struggled on and got the lifeboat afloat with their second attempt.

On 11 February 1974, the wind was at hurricane force and there was a badly injured man on board the ship *Merc Texco* who needed to be brought ashore. So big were the waves breaking on the beach that the launchers had to be roped together as they placed the skids, for fear they would be washed away. When they reached the water's edge the lifeboat became stuck in the shingle and two huge waves broached her. These were major problems for the launchers and the crew, but the coxswain, using his skill and working hard, managed to set the lifeboat seawards and in the direction of the casualty. More skilful handling was needed when the lifeboat reached the ship, but eventually the injured man was placed safely aboard the lifeboat and taken as quickly as possible to medical help. All the launchers were exhausted but happy that there had been a successful outcome to their efforts. In recognition that these were the worst beach conditions ever experienced at Dungeness, the launchers again received Thanks on Vellum.

One of the women launchers on both these occasions was Doris Tart, who gave forty-four years' service as a launcher. Doris was born Doris Oiller and chose Ben Tart as her husband, creating a link between the two main families of Dungeness. Both families have long linkages with the service and have held many positions of responsibility on the lifeboat. Ben was no exception, and it was he who was coxswain in 1974. It is said that the Tarts and Oillers have lifeboating in their blood. From her earliest years, Doris learned what was expected of Dungeness women – hardly surprising, since she was surrounded by female relatives who gave their heart and soul to supporting their men folk on the crew. Doris's mother-in-law, Ellen, and her aunt, Madge, were awarded the RNLI Gold Badge in 1954 – both had given service for over fifty years.

Like all the women, Doris's greatest fears were for the crew's safety. She was particularly concerned when the lifeboat was coming ashore after picking up the injured man from the *Merc Texco*: 'When they first came back from there I didn't want them to come ashore. I thought it was too rough. The sea was tremendous.'

Doris was awarded a Gold Badge on her retirement in 1979. Throughout her life she had collected many RNLI artefacts and these she gave to the lifeboat gallery in the Historic Dockyard at Chatham, where they are now on display. When Doris Tart died in 2007, aged eighty-five, the RNLI said goodbye to the last 'lady launcher'.

Launching the lifeboats today

The RNLI still has many women launchers, now known as Shore Crew – at the time of publication they number approximately eighty-two. Women are volunteering for Shore Crew in all parts of the country, although the greatest proportion is in the south-east. Over the past five years, there has been a steady growth in the number of women coming forward to do this essential work. The average age for women Shore Crew is thirty-six years, which is a little older than that of women volunteering for lifeboat crew or to be a lifeguard.

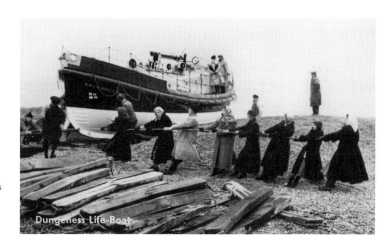

Postcard of Dungeness women launchers in 1950. (Iain Booth postcard collection)

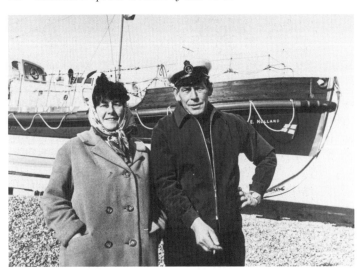

Doris and Ben Tart:
Doris was the last 'lady
launcher' of the RNLI.
(*Kent Messenger*)

Today lifeboat launching takes advantage of the technology and pulling power of tractors and all-terrain vehicles rather than human muscle. There is a real requirement for skill, knowledge and good judgement when using this heavy equipment in challenging coastal environments, often in adverse weather – launching lifeboats is still potentially a dangerous undertaking. In line with all other operational policies, Shore Crew must undertake structured training before being allowed to use the equipment.

Launching and recovering lifeboats is as essential a part of saving life at sea as ever it was, and the women who give their commitment to a lifeboat station to do this are key to an effective service. Operating in very different parts of our coastline, women follow the great tradition of female lifeboat launchers. Over the years, the RNLI has invested in sophisticated technology to make launching lifeboats quicker, safer and less dependent on pure physical strength. Even so, the skill required in the operation of a lifeboat launch should never be underestimated. If something is done incorrectly, there is the risk of serious injury to the launchers. A delay in launching may also jeopardise the whole rescue, which could result in lives being lost.

Representing the female launchers of the twenty-first century, four women from different parts of the coast speak of their experience today.

Trisha Bradford, St Ives

Trisha Bradford is the daughter of St Ives coxswain Tommy Cocking, and grew up with lifeboating at the very heart of family life. As a child, she experienced all the lifestyle restrictions of having a father who had to be near to the boathouse and accepted that this was the way of things. She felt sadness when he could not visit her in hospital but understood about his commitment and respected what he stood for. Mostly she was unafraid, but can recall occasions on which there was a shout when the wind was shaking the house, and she realised that half her family were out in an open lifeboat that did only seven knots. She took heart from her mother who seemed not to bat an eyelid that her husband was in danger, and yet again patiently waited for his return.

Trisha Bradford, launcher at
St Ives Lifeboat Station.

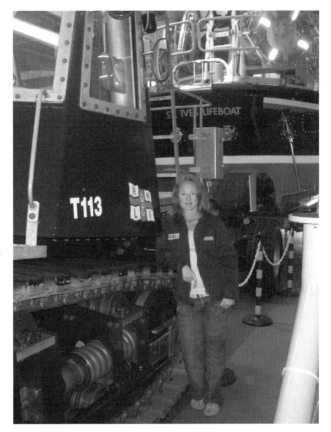

It was when Trisha was a teenager that she first asked her father if she could have a go on the tractor. He said no. Undaunted, Trisha contin-ued to ask and ask but always got the same answer. Trisha now knows that he said no because he was concerned that yet another member of the family would be commit-ted to the demands of being ever available for a lifeboat launch. She recalls him saying 'Murderers don't get this sen-tence!' Eventually there came a time when Tommy was short of tractor drivers and the Lifeboat Inspector, sens-ing Trisha's frustration, asked why she did not drive. An explanation was given, but a week later her father offered her the chance. Having yearned for it for so long, Trisha now felt nervous – this was for real.

The training completed, the day came for her to take her test. Absolutely no pressure on Trisha as the whole town knew what was happening. 'I thought I would die,' she recalls. Unsurprisingly she passed and has now been driving the tractor for seven years. It has fulfilled her every expectation: 'It's infectious, the more you get called, the more you want to get called. You know there is some poor soul in trouble and you want to help.' Once the station had fourteen calls in ten days, and Trisha recalls being out until 2a.m. on a number of occasions. This could be a problem for a mother with young children, but Trisha knows they love the fact that their Mum drives the tractor and they do all they can to help when her pager goes off. She has put various systems in place for childcare depending on the time of day; sometimes family and sometimes friends. Trisha is confident that in her community her children will be well looked after while she launches and recovers the lifeboat.

Being a Shore Helper brings many challenges, many laughs, some tears and many fulfil-ments. Trisha is certain that being a woman does not detract from her ability to be a true member of and make a full contribution to the team. As 'just one of the blokes', she knows that she would do anything for each of them and she could turn for help to anyone. She knows she is fortunate to have a husband who understands and copes with the disruptions that occur, but as he is a diver, he knows how important it is to have the RNLI always ready to come to the rescue.

Rianne Smith and Kate Callanan, Baltimore

The nicknames given to the women launchers at Baltimore Lifeboat Station might be regarded as more than cheeky by some, but for Rianne, Kate and Gwen (no longer on the team), it was great fun. They were called 'Slip Bitch', 'Winch Wench' and 'Hooker'.

The names neatly capture the individual roles undertaken while launching the Tyne class lifeboat down the slipway and into the sea. Anyone who has ever seen the launch of an all-weather lifeboat fourteen metres long and weighing twenty-five tonnes down a slipway will appreciate what great skill is required for this operation. A minimum of three people are needed.

Neither Rianne nor Kate was born in Baltimore, but both fell in love with the place and resolved to live there. Rianne, a Dutch national, runs a diving business with her husband Jerry, who is 2nd mechanic in the lifeboat crew. Kate enjoyed childhood holidays in Baltimore and remembers collecting for the lifeboat on August bank holidays. She is currently working as a wedding and events coordinator and is married to Mícheál who, with his brother, is third generation lifeboat crew.

Rianne remembers driving Jerry to the station when his pager went off and often getting involved with launching when they were short of helpers. In 1998 she decided to join officially. Then she was the only woman on the crew, but not deterred, she attended training courses and enjoyed the camaraderie. Kate uses the word 'inevitable' to describe how she became a lifeboat launcher. She would hear Mícheál's pager go off in the night and after he vanished to the boathouse, she would find herself awake and waiting anxiously. She thought she would like to get involved herself, but felt she was not cut out to join the crew. Mícheál suggested she try the slip crew, and six years later she knows that was the right decision.

The work of the slip crew is an essential element of a lifeboat service; not just in launching the lifeboat, but also in the less dramatic process of recovering it afterwards. No job is complete until the boat is housed, washed, refuelled and ready for service. Kate describes the process:

> Regardless of the time of day or night, buckets of soapy water and sponges in hand, the crew and slip crew wash the boat from top to bottom! Recently, there was a call out and the boat launched at 1.50a.m. They didn't return to the station until 2.30p.m. Although the crew were tired not one of the crew that had been out on the call left the boathouse before the washdown and refuelling was complete. This in my mind is true testament to the total commitment of the lifeboat team we have here in Baltimore.

Rianne confirms that they are essentially one team with a special bond made by their mutual dedication to saving lives. Both she and Kate feel huge respect for the crew who go out in all weathers and whose courage is a constant source of motivation when the call to launch the lifeboat comes.

Rianne remembers launching the lifeboat in all kinds of clothing: wetsuit, bikini, evening dress and high heels – the need for a lifeboat launch rarely comes at a convenient time and sometimes there is no time to change into their protective kit, comprising overalls and weatherproof gear. This is far from ideal, because launching, as well as being physically

Theresa Shammon and Michelle
Stewardson – Ramsey lifeboat launchers.

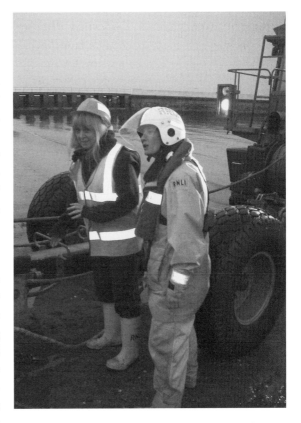

hard work – dragging ropes, steel
hooks and wires, opening heavy
sliding doors – is also very dirty, as
everything is covered in grease. The
one thing she and Kate guard carefully are their precious steel-capped
yellow wellies – they wear sizes four
and five, whereas some of the men
need size fourteen or fifteen boots!

Theresa Shammon, Ramsey

Theresa just happened to be watching a practice launch of the Ramsey
lifeboat when someone shouted to
her: 'Here pull this!' The next thing
she knew she was pulling like mad
at a rope and helping the crew to
move the heavy Mersey class lifeboat out of the boathouse, across a
stretch of beach and into the sea. So
began her involvement as a launcher – a volunteer commitment that has continued for
eighteen years.

When Coxswain Jimmy Kinnin realised that she had come back to help with launching on several occasions he said: 'I don't know why you don't join the crew.' The idea was
attractive to Theresa – a marine scientist who loves the sea. Her husband, Kim, was already
on the crew. Much to her disappointment her eyesight prevented her from joining the
boat crew, so she made a conscious decision to make her contribution on the shore crew.
Now she is one of two head launchers at the station and she is qualified to drive the tractor. Additionally she is the Station Press Officer. It is quite a commitment but, as Theresa
observes, the RNLI relies on some people giving money and others giving their time.

At Ramsey there are strong bonds between the boat crew, who must actively help with
launching and recovery, and the shore crew. Theresa remains behind but her thoughts stay
with the lifeboat throughout the service. Sometimes it is only afterwards that she allows
herself to think about the implications of the danger involved.

Theresa's view that she gets as much back as she gives from her volunteer support is
echoed by fellow crew member Michelle Stewardson, who has been on the boat crew for
almost eight years. For Michelle, a psychiatric social worker, it feels good to do something
completely different from normal work, while pushing yourself beyond your comfort zone.
She considers that one of the great achievements of the RNLI is that, at every lifeboat station, they bring together a disparate group of individuals and form them into an effective
team, which goes on to quite remarkable achievements.

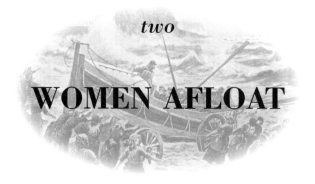

two

WOMEN AFLOAT

Following tradition

Having women to launch lifeboats was entirely acceptable to the early RNLI lifeboat crews, but involving women in a rescue stopped as soon as the lifeboat was afloat. There was no question of them joining the men as crew because traditional wisdom held that having women onboard made the sea angry and was an omen for bad luck. Operating in such a dangerous environment meant that mariners and fishermen were at best conservative and at worst superstitious. Their beliefs placed emphasis on the relatively small matters they could control, as compared with the unpredictable sea, which they could not. As most lifeboat crew had a maritime or fishing background, the female role was clearly understood by both sexes.

Grace Darling is often misrepresented as being a member of a lifeboat crew, but she was not. At his request she assisted her father to rescue people shipwrecked on one of the Farne Islands where William Darling was a lighthouse keeper. For her great bravery, she was awarded a medal by the RNLI (page 47). It was the first to be presented to a woman, and the RNLI is proud to celebrate her achievements at the Grace Darling Museum, but she was never a member of a lifeboat crew.

It was not until 1969 that the RNLI accepted its first woman crew member; in 2009 there were 374. This represents 8 per cent of all RNLI crew. Seventy-three per cent of the 235 lifeboat stations have women on their crew. Ireland has the largest number of women crew, followed by the West Country. There is a fairly even spread of women crew between the ages of eighteen to twenty-four, twenty-five to thirty-four, and thirty-five to forty-nine.

The introduction of inshore lifeboats into the fleet in the 1960s acted as a catalyst to break the long tradition of all male crews. Women were first accepted to crew these lighter, more manoeuvrable craft, and as they proved their competence, it was only a matter of time before women joined all-weather lifeboat crews.

Changing the tradition

Elizabeth Hostvedt – first woman on an inshore lifeboat crew

Elizabeth, who had a Norwegian father and Scots mother, was in 1967 among the first nine girls accepted at Atlantic College in South Wales. To encourage their involvement in the local community, all students were required to choose from a range of social service activities. Elizabeth elected to join the crew of the lifeboat station at the College after it became clear that the beach rescue team – her first choice – was not keen to have girls. Quickly she realised that a much higher level of technical skill was required in the lifeboat as well as much more team collaboration, and this certainly played to her strengths. She followed the very thorough training and on completion her name was among those sent to RNLI HQ for registration as lifeboat crew.

There has been something of an urban myth about whether officials at HQ realised at this stage that Elizabeth was female, but having looked at the original ledger, I can confirm that her full name is recorded – so it was most definitely known. Once the news got out, there was a lot of media interest in this great break with tradition. Elizabeth remembers it as good fun and she enjoyed meeting Chay Blyth and John Ridgeway at the Boat Show, and being interviewed by Jack de Manio on the radio. Her mother proudly collected all the newspaper clippings, including the ones which Elizabeth says were deliberately taken to show off her legs!

Looking back, Elizabeth realises that she was involved with the RNLI at a very special time, when there was a huge impetus to develop lighter, stronger boats. Her experience at sea was exciting and she cannot remember feeling fear, although sometimes recovering the lifeboat onto the trolley was 'hairy'. She had a healthy respect for the sea and a desire to help people in trouble. Elizabeth is quite certain that her time on the lifeboat crew made her grow up and helped her to understand how people function in a team.

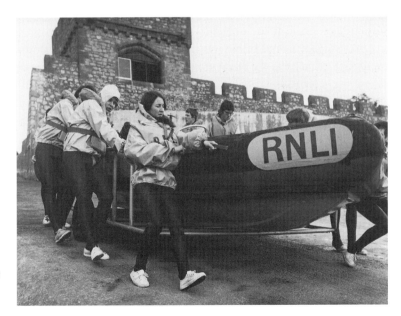

Elizabeth Hostvedt of Atlantic College; first woman inshore lifeboat crew member.

Elizabeth now lives in England with her husband, son and daughter and works as a land-scape gardener.

Frances Glody – first woman on an all-weather lifeboat crew

In 1981, when Frances Glody was accepted at Dunmore East Lifeboat Station to crew on the Waveney class lifeboat *St Patrick*, Ireland already had three women crewing inshore life-boats. Frances was the first woman crew member on an offshore (now termed all-weather) crew.

Becoming the first ever woman all-weather crew member was a second 'first' for Frances. She had already caused something of a stir when, at just twenty years old, she was appointed to the post of Pilot Station Master at Dunmore East. Taking over from her father who had just retired, she was following three generations of Glody men who had held the post. She was not only the first Glody woman to take responsibility for guiding ships into the har-bours of Waterford and New Ross, she was also the first woman in Ireland ever to be Pilot Station Master.

Frances readily acknowledges her passion for the sea and recalls how her father had hoped to cure her by taking her out in very rough conditions with the aim of making her seasick. He hoped that the misery of being sick might focus her attention towards what he felt to be more feminine interests. She was not seasick and never has been since. His plan had failed and although Frances loves to crochet, her heart is locked into the sea and ships. She took it as quite natural that her two brothers, Patrick and Brendan, were members of the local lifeboat crew, but never considered that she might join herself: 'I used to look at the crew members in their oilskins going out to battle against the elements. But in the wildest flight of my imagination I never thought I'd be out there one day with them.'

It was Frances's concern to do her Pilot job well, which triggered a chain of events that led to her joining the crew. The lifeboat crew were doing an RNLI radio course delivered in a caravan at the lifeboat station and, with the coxswain's agreement, Frances joined her brothers so that she could brush up on her radio procedure skills. At the end of the six-week course, she took the exam and passed – as did all the other nine crew.

This called for a celebration, and it was at the Ocean Hotel that Frances heard Coxswain Stephen Whittle say to the Lifeboat Inspector, Tony Course: 'If I was ever stuck for a member I'd ask her, she knows it all.' Frances recalls the moment when the Inspector turned to her

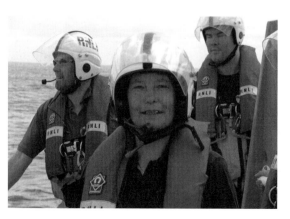

and said: 'Why not, why don't you apply?' She thought he was 'only messing', but the following morn-ing he gave her an application form. 'I was amazed and astonished,' she says. After a stiff medical in Dublin, the official word came from RNLI HQ – miles away in Dorset – that she had been accepted.

Frances Glody of Dunmore East; first woman all-weather lifeboat crew member.

Making this piece of RNLI history brought considerable media attention in the early 1980s. Frances has a scrapbook of the newspaper cuttings which carry headlines to announce the startling fact that a woman was to be doing what only men had done for over 150 years: 'The only girl in a lifeboat' (*Irish Press*); 'A new darling of the sea set sail with our lifeboat heroes' (*Daily Mail*); 'A Girl's Touch' (*Annabel*); 'Frances to the Rescue' (*Mail on Sunday*). At the time this was all exciting for her, but Frances recalls that as she got older, she was rather embarrassed by the attention, knowing that she was just one of a 'great team'.

Interest focused on whether a woman could do what traditionally it was believed only men could achieve. Frances fielded the questions with typical lifeboat crew modesty, saying:

> I don't feel it's different for me because I'm a woman. I know the sea and I have the qualifica-
> tions to do the job … I don't see lifeboat work as being a brave job to do. You don't do a job
> like that from bravery. I wouldn't say I'm courageous, but I think the greatest satisfaction is the
> thought that some day you will be able to save a life.

Not every shout has a happy ending, though, and Frances remembers vividly the first dead body she had to deal with: 'It was the body of a child and later I was afraid to go to bed and sleep in case I would dream of it. Fortunately, I didn't.' After hundreds of shouts, Frances retired from the crew when she reached her fiftieth birthday, and looks back with pride on 'being a lifeboat man – it was a very worthwhile and satisfying use of my time'.

Women crew in the twenty-first century

To some it is a matter of great surprise to learn that the RNLI has so many women serving on lifeboat crews; the most common preconception is that women are not strong enough to undertake the arduous work required. Some people have a deeply embedded stereotype of the big, brave, bearded lifeboat man, and it is a hard one to break. Others rejoice in the role that women are now fulfilling at the sharp end of saving lives at sea and feel that the RNLI should give more publicity to their women lifeboat crew. Another view is that what the women do is so normal and natural that there should be no distinction made – and certainly no fuss. At the very end of the opinion spectrum there are reminders that women wanted equality, so should expect no special attention.

In the forty years since a woman was first accepted on a lifeboat crew, hundreds of women have followed and given their serious commitment to following the accepted operational requirements and standards that the RNLI lays down for all crew. They have completed the training requirements, attended regular practice, carried a pager and responded to it twenty-four hours a day, 365 days a year, risked their lives, left their families to worry until their safe return, and acted as good ambassadors for the RNLI. None of this is in any way different from what the men of the crews do.

For many women, though, the challenges of coming into a traditional service have been considerable, and it is a tribute to their determination and desire to succeed that so many have established themselves as both competent and respected. There are too many women crew for all to contribute to this book – those who have volunteered are therefore representative voices for the 374 women currently serving. They speak of why and how they joined; what their experience has been; and what being a woman of the RNLI means to them.

Karolyn Rath, Clogher Head

Having a station mechanic father, lifeboating has always been a part of Karolyn's life. She has many childhood memories of dinners half eaten and cups of tea left to go cold when her father abandoned the house to race to the lifeboat. A particularly poignant memory was watching the rescue of an overturned yacht in the harbour and being so impressed by the way in which the coxswain manoeuvred the lifeboat. There was the happy day in 1993 when the crew brought their new Mersey class lifeboat to Clogher Head. The whole village was festooned with posters and banners to welcome the lifeboat and children were given a day off school. Karolyn understood on that day just how valued the lifeboat service is in her community.

It was thought quite natural for her brother to join the crew, but when, in 2001, Karolyn volunteered, the reaction was somewhat different. She knew that her father would be a hard taskmaster – his belief was that you gave all or nothing to the lifeboat. While the men on the crew were helpful, Karolyn knew they were watching to see if she was tough enough. The thought seemed to be that she might last for a couple of shouts and that would be it. She recalls being treated no differently from any other starter. The great thing was to learn how to take the jokes and to give them back – crew humour is one of the things that she now enjoys and values.

Nine years later, Karolyn has more than proved that she is tough enough, but she acknowledges that there are times when it is hard. She has memories of one shout when, after a long, fruitless search for a man overboard, they had to walk away. For a long time she could not stop thinking about the body out there.

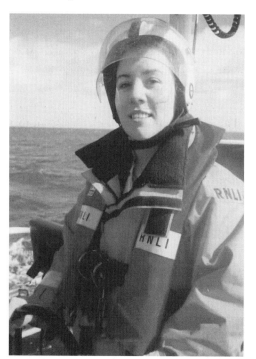

Karolyn is a primary school teacher and finds that she can use her lifeboat experience as a great resource for teaching. She uses stories and visits to the boathouse as a means of experiencing something very different from their everyday lives. Her hope is that the children may be encouraged to become involved. For her, being involved is a source of great pride; to be following the family tradition and to be giving something to her community. Once the prospect of being winched up into a helicopter seemed impossible – but not now!

Karolyn Rath of Clogher Head lifeboat crew.

Cath Fox, Southwold

Cath joined in 1999, having been encouraged by the crew to volunteer. Growing up in Lancashire and having family holidays at Abersoch, she had always loved the sea and had much sailing experience. She had also gained her powerboat instructor qualification. Moving to Southwold to take up a teaching post with nine- to thirteen-year-old children, Cath was impressed with the strong community spirit there and she wanted to be a part of it. Back in Lancashire, her parents, both supporters of the RNLI, were delighted with the news of Cath's involvement at Southwold – her mother is a regular collector in Preston.

For a while, Cath was one of three women on the crew and recalls how positive everyone was towards her. She immediately felt a part of the team and as the years have passed, with a growing number of experiences shared, she feels this even more strongly. There was the time when they were called out to two little girls desperately clinging on to the harbour wall, their mother doing all she could to hold them up. How grateful they were, as was their father, who later wrote thanking the crew. An early morning shout to go to the aid of a fisherman who had been washed off the beach in a huge tidal surge brought a rescue attempt in enormous rolling waves. In a long search involving Lowestoft and Cromer lifeboats as well as a helicopter, the Southwold lifeboat tried to find the man in the water. Cath operated the radio for five hours and remembers feeling deaf for hours afterwards. Sadly the man was not found and his body was washed ashore two weeks later.

There was another occasion when the same lifeboats and a helicopter were scrambled because a signal from an EPIRB (Emergency Position Indicating Radio Beacon) had been received. Conditions were particularly difficult because of the thick fog. Cath was onboard the Southwold lifeboat which was tasked to search close to the beach. For three hours they followed a search pattern up and down, hardly able to see a thing through the fog, but finding nothing. The signal from the EPIRB should have led them straight to the casualty, but the helicopter reported difficulty in getting a fix – which was hardly surprising when it was later discovered that the EPIRB had accidentally gone off while on a wardrobe shelf in the middle of the town! The crews salvaged the situation by agreeing that it was a very good – albeit expensive – training exercise for searching in fog.

For Cath, lifeboating is a way of life – a great way of life that enables her to follow her family tradition of giving community service. The RNLI is held in such high esteem that at school she notices that the children look at lifeboat crew in a slightly different way. Something must have rubbed off because now some of the crew are her ex-pupils. That is something else that she finds so very good about the RNLI – that crew members come from all walks of life and very successfully form a team that goes on to achieve amazing things.

Pauline Dunleavy, Kilrush

Pauline comes from a farming background and owns a craft shop, but was interested to hear that the RNLI had plans to set up a new lifeboat station at Kilrush. There was no lifeboat on the Shannon estuary and one was needed to provide cover for these busy waters. A public meeting was called and Pauline went with a friend, thinking that maybe she would give a hand by joining the committee. After listening to an RNLI representative urging people to volunteer for crew, the friend persuaded Pauline that they should both sign up.

Pauline surprised herself by saying yes, knowing that she was 'no good on the water' and ironically, the friend never joined.

So from day one of this new station, Pauline has been deeply involved and is now the senior helm and Lifeboat Training Officer; more recently she has been appointed Lifeboat Press Officer. From the start she had fun, enjoying the camaraderie of the crew who were 'a lovely bunch of guys' – no other women volunteered in the early days. While Pauline loves giving service to her community, she knows how the lifeboat service is valued locally. A friendly wave is always given to a car that carries lifeboat crew stickers.

Carrying a pager was a completely new experience and for the first few shouts took her by surprise when it went off, especially at night. Once when fast asleep she did not hear it, but her husband did. 'Get up, your man is talking to you,' he said. Pauline knows that he was worried about her safety and waited by the window of their kitchen anxiously for the lifeboat to return. She says this only lasted for the first three or four shouts and then it was he who often slept through the pager calls.

Of all the shouts she has done, Pauline remembers one when she and her crew unquestionably saved a man's life because they were able to provide first aid with great competence. Curiously, it occurred four days after an RNLI first-aid trainer had been at the station introducing a new checklist that was to be invaluable for the crew in helping the casualty. In foggy conditions a French sailor had been hit hard on the head by the boom. When the lifeboat arrived they found he was concussed and bleeding from an ear. The crew followed the recently learned procedure and radioed for an airlift. Later they were advised that the man had been within ten minutes of losing his life.

Pauline is keen to support women to become lifeboat crew and recognises that it is difficult for those who have babies and young children. She certainly gives short shrift to anyone who thinks women are not up to the job.

Now looking forward to the arrival of a new Atlantic 85 lifeboat in 2010, Pauline is quick to acknowledge not just the 'superb crew' at Kilrush, but also the people who worked so hard to fundraise and set up the station. She points to two women she admires, Dr Kathleen Ryan and Mrs Gwen Glynn, who spent hours standing on corners with collecting boxes and gives thanks for the generosity of the public.

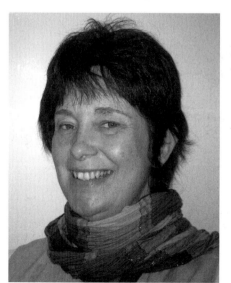

Carolyn Newlands, Helensburgh

Carolyn's first attempt to join the lifeboat crew at Helensburgh was not well received. In fact she was actually told that the RNLI did not accept female volunteers to serve as crew members. This was in 1986, when there were already quite a number of women serving on crews. As a keen sailor, Carolyn did not allow this rejection to cloud her understanding of the value of

Pauline Dunleavy of Kilrush lifeboat crew.

the RNLI, and she jumped at the chance when approached the following year with the question: 'Are you still interested to join the crew?' Fortunately, someone, somewhere had done some rethinking!

Her job as office manageress/company secretary for a marine civil engineering company was based in an office just fifty yards from the lifeboat station, and she already knew many of the crew who accepted her straight away. After three months' training she was assessed by the Divisional Inspector who accepted her as Helensburgh's first female crew member. Another first for Carolyn was when a few years later she became the first woman helm in the whole of Scotland. At this time she also took on the role of station trainer and really enjoyed passing on her knowledge and experience to new volunteers. By now she was not the only woman on the crew, as she had helped to enrol two others.

The protective clothing worn by all crew is very effective camouflage and often it is not until the helmet is removed that the sex of the wearer is revealed. For Carolyn while on a rescue to a broken-down yacht with four people on board, it was when she took her gloves off that she heard surprise in their voices: 'It's a woman!' They were then intrigued by how she managed to keep her nails so long and painted. Carolyn is much amused by this and can list other funny incidents related to being a woman on a lifeboat crew:

> On a long shout in an Atlantic 21 with no facilities, not even a bucket, … scattering ashes when the wind changes, not holding on when the helm of the boat puts on full throttle from standstill to 30 knots … splash!! Going up and down on a helicopter winch wire that is not designed for the female figure, changing out of your best frock with half a dozen pairs of male eyes watching, looking like you forgot to take your makeup off when you went to bed when you return from a shout, and as for the bad hair days …

For Carolyn, there are particular shouts that make it all worthwhile. Of the 111 she has been actively involved in, she recalls going to a capsized dinghy, arriving forty minutes after

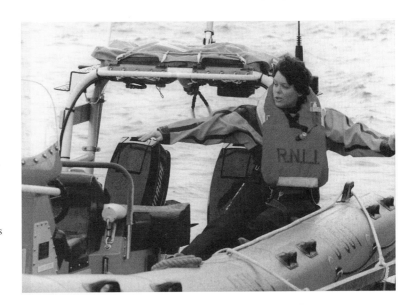

Carolyn Newlands of Helensburgh in the Atlantic 75 lifeboat *Gladys Winifred Tiffney*.

it had capsized to find three men in the water in the Gareloch. The crew got all three into the lifeboat and ashore at a local boatyard and kept them warm until the ambulance arrived. She says: 'This kind of shout makes you feel very good about yourself as you have actually saved life at sea.'

Vivian Bailey, Loch Ness

A home in the Highlands of Scotland is not the most promising location for an aspiring crew member, but when in 2008 the RNLI established the first inland lifeboat station in Scotland on Loch Ness, Vivian decided to go for it. So did her partner, Martin Douglas, who volunteered at the same time.

Having a mother who was a very positive role model for equality had always convinced Vivian that she could do pretty much anything she set her mind to. Looking back to when she was making the decision to join the crew, Vivian remembers how important the support of her youngest son, a teenager, was to her. He was adamant that neither she nor Martin should worry if he were left at home on his own because of a shout. For him, it was more important that they were out saving lives. There was nothing but encouragement from the rest of the crew. As it was a brand new station there were no preconceptions and women were accepted very naturally. On the crew at Loch Ness there are now three women and another in the process of joining.

Vivian believes she has received excellent training and is convinced that when she and the crew were involved in the challenging rescue of a young girl with a suspected spinal injury, the training kicked in automatically to ensure that everyone functioned as an effective team. When the lifeboat arrived, the casualty, who had been thrown off a 'doughnut' being towed at speed, was in the water being supported by two girls who happened to be lifeguards at the local swimming pool. The loch water was very cold and all three were verging on hypothermic. One of the crew got into the water to replace one of the girls while Vivian prepared the stretcher in readiness for the helicopter that had been summoned. The winch was completed smoothly and when the young girl reached hospital she was diagnosed with three spinal fractures – happily she has since recovered well. A witness on the shore was convinced it was an exercise because everything had been done in textbook style!

As a keen sailor and canoeist, Vivian has always known that, should she get into trouble, she could rely on the RNLI. Now she is the one providing that reassurance for others. As a geography teacher she is able to bring the RNLI into her lessons and explain why it is that the crews are willing to volunteer to save lives. In fact, any 'spare' time has been pretty much volunteered away, both in her work as an education speaker and as the Loch Ness Coordinator for the Future Crew Project, which aims to train young people to take one of the many possible volunteer roles in the RNLI. Vivian is especially proud that one of the first graduates from the scheme is a female from Loch Ness station who is now applying to join the crew.

Sharon Gozna, Rye Harbour

Sharon's first experience of the lifeboat community was through her husband, Mark, who joined the Rye Harbour crew in 2005. Interested in what he had become involved with,

Sharon Gozna of Rye Harbour with her now late husband Mark.

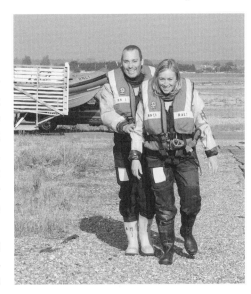

she went to the social events, got to know everyone, and quickly realised what great people they were. She could see that there were 'terrific characters' in the team and that they had a great deal of fun, as well as working very hard and facing danger together. Sharon decided this was definitely for her, volunteered, and threw herself into the training.

Now she and Mark were learning together and it was a very happy experience. One that was sadly not to last because the cancer he had beaten eight years previously returned. Mark started high-dose chemotherapy and radiotherapy, but the treatment was not successful and he died in March 2008. Heartbroken, Sharon had no idea just how much her Rye Harbour friends were going to help her:

> I can honestly say that that I don't know how I would have coped without the incredible and unfaltering support I got from the crew and all at the station. They gave him a full RNLI funeral and were right by my side on the boat with me to scatter Mark's ashes at sea. They became like a family to me and they encouraged me to continue my training to become a full crew member. I threw myself into it like never before, trained with all of them on the station, went on the five-day course at Poole and came back fully qualified.

Sharon, who works in interior design, is convinced that apart from marrying Mark, joining a lifeboat crew is the best thing she has ever done. RNLI family values helped her manage bereavement and nurtured her self-confidence to believe that she had something of her own to offer others. She is now training to become a helm and, while accepting that she has her work cut out to achieve this, she is determined to give it her best shot.

When asked what the RNLI has given her, she answered: 'A whole sense of humour, a sense of purpose and a sense of protection.' While not claiming to be a spiritual person, she is convinced that she can't help but think she was introduced to the crew for a reason.

Nicki Wood, Sheerness

In 2002, Nicki presented her husband, David, with an ultimatum – they must either move to Sheerness or to St Ives. Why? So that Nicki could join the crew at one of those lifeboat stations. They were living in Rainham, Kent, so David chose Sheerness as being the nearer by far. Twelve weeks later they moved, and the first thing Nicki did was to speak to the coxswain about joining the crew. In describing the background to these dramatic events, Nicki explains that as a child she 'fell in love' with the lifeboat when holidaying in St Ives. This enduring passion would lead to the ultimatum.

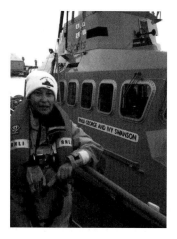

Nicki Wood of Sheerness with Trent class lifeboat *George and Ivy Swanson.*

A keen swimmer, she became a volunteer lifeguard while still at school. This involved patrolling the beach on the Isle of Sheppey where, some years later, when her children were older, she joined the Auxiliary Coastguard. She was amazed to find there was a lifeboat at Sheerness and decided it might after all be possible to make her dream come true. She knew she did not have much boating experience and was slightly built, but her enthusiasm was very strong.

There were no other women on the crew, but the coxswain was welcoming and made it clear that 'as long as she did the same as everyone else there would be no problems'. Some of the crew were not so sure. Nicki describes the silences she encountered in the early days as 'frosty'. These lasted for several months, but she followed the advice given by the coxswain, showing that she was prepared to do exactly what they did. When the leg pulling started she knew she was making progress. Nicki did not mind and did her bit to get her own back. What was important to her was that she had no special treatment and she is adamant that this is the only way to make it work – women should not expect to be treated differently. Everyone in their team takes their turn with the less attractive jobs, including cleaning the boathouse and making the tea.

Her first shout as helm was special and nerve-wracking. It was to two people in the water near the Sheerness outfall. The coastguard rescued one and Nicki and crew brought the lifeboat alongside just in time as the other was slipping under the water. On that day she truly felt that she had made a difference, and it confirmed her conviction that joining the lifeboat crew is the most important thing she has done in her life. In fact, she feels that it has been her destiny since she was a small child. After the difficult start she now says emphatically: 'The crew are my best friends. I would trust them with my life. We have such a laugh, even in the most difficult situations. Life without the boat would be unimaginable.'

And her family uprooted to make all this possible? Nicki says they understand, although not quite so much when her pager went off on Christmas Eve and she did not return until the early hours of Christmas Day!

Eleanor Hooker, Lough Derg

'It didn't strike us as unusual – we all sailed and some worked on the water or at the local boatyard.' Eleanor speaks for the six women who volunteered in 2004 to join the crew of a lifeboat station to be established on Lough Derg, the second largest lake in the Republic of Ireland.

What they did feel was a sense of honour to be involved in something as noble as saving lives. Add to this the opportunity of giving something back to their community and the certainty of receiving excellent training from the RNLI, and the decision to join up was an easy one. Eleanor, with a nursing background and currently studying for her MPhil at Trinity College, Dublin is now the helm, as well as Station Press Officer. Being on the crew means so much to her that she dreads the day she is too old to crew: 'I have threatened to motorise my Zimmer frame so I can make it to the station in my dotage!'

While her family give her much support, there is some amusement about how she looks in her protective gear. Seeing Eleanor in it for the first time, her sister called her Buzz Lightyear and yelled 'To infinity and beyond!' Her husband is no more complimentary, but Eleanor says it is the only outfit of which she will allow him to say: 'Honey, your bum does look big in that!'

Eleanor has noticed that women on board casualty vessels more rapidly set up a rapport with their female rescuers, whilst men can sometimes be sullen – she suggests perhaps because being rescued by a woman increases their mortification. Her first shout as helm was, she recalls, a baptism of fire. In gale force 7/gusting 8 winds, seven people on holiday from Germany had gone aground in a cruiser. When another cruiser went aground, she was the helm on the first all-female shout. As the lifeboat approached, they heard a small boy's voice say 'Daddy, daddy, we're OK, the lifeboat's here,' shortly followed by 'Daddy, daddy, they are all women!' To which Eleanor retorted: 'Will you wait then till we go back and find some men?' Afterwards all the crew laughed, but they knew they had done a good job in very trying conditions.

People are frequently very afraid when they find themselves in danger at sea, which Eleanor readily recognises and responds to:

> When we go to a vessel in distress, fear is a physical thing which prowls the deck, which taunts the people on the vessel. When we climb aboard, crack a joke, smile, appear confident, we take fear away and give people the confidence that we are going to take them home safe and sound. That feeling of being able to help, to take people away from the nightmare they find themselves in, is fantastic.

Nora Flanagan, Arranmore

What does a keen crew member do when the dreaded day comes to retire? There are so many other ways to continue to play an active part in the RNLI. If you are Nora Flanagan, you grab them …

As the first women on the Arranmore lifeboat crew, Nora attracted quite a bit of local press interest and felt she had become a 'novelty act'. She recalls that giving interviews was the most frightening part of being a lifeboat crew member, and marvels that she is now the Station Press Officer.

Nora describes Arranmore as paradise, and for that reason returned to live there with her husband and children after a period nursing in London where she had hoped 'to find her fortune'. Memories of her happy childhood on the island convinced her that the best fortune was to be found on the west coast of County Donegal. Growing up on Arranmore, and with the lifeboat anchored practically outside her front door, with the constant danger of the sea well known to her, she admits to not having taken very much notice of the lifeboat – until she attended an RNLI first-aid course at the lifeboat station at which members of the public were welcome. It was a good course, Nora remembers, and maybe it was the enthusiasm of the instructor for the RNLI that prompted her to volunteer herself when at the end of the evening the mechanic asked if anyone was interested to join the crew.

Everyone was amazed – this was not what was expected of a woman. Seeing the reaction, Nora thought she would hear no more, but the mechanic was true to his word and invited her on the next exercise. Having donned the protective gear, she boarded the lifeboat and was thrilled by its sheer power and speed as they set off. Soon she overheard one of the crew say to the coxswain, 'Take her round the island at full speed and that will make her sick'. A bad error of judgement, says Nora: 'It was just the thing I needed to convince me that this was exactly what I wanted to be doing – and I wasn't sick!'

Her first shout left her feeling dejected, as hours of searching for a fisherman overboard brought no result and she had felt pretty useless throughout. Fortunately she did not hand in her pager, as she promised herself she would, because on the next shout – which came the very same day – she was able to make a difference. Her nursing skills were vital in helping the casualty to start breathing again. On returning to work at the local day centre, Nora realised that everybody on the crew has a role to play, whatever the level and type of their experience, and she served on the crew for seven years. The Arranmore lifeboat performs many medical evacuations from the island, often women in labour, and many have said how reassured they have been to have a nurse within the crew.

The buzz she gets now that she is no longer on the crew comes from making people aware of the work the crew do and their dedication to saving lives: 'despite their modesty, the crews appreciate getting the recognition they deserve and every story serves to heighten the profile of the lifeboat service.'

Toilet issues!

A sensitive subject maybe, but a very practical concern for all aboard a lifeboat for hours on end. For women, there are real challenges. Firstly, because the female anatomy is less conducive to an 'al fresco' wee than the male. Secondly, because women are usually in the minority on a lifeboat and there can be sensitivities about when and how to do the necessary.

Coxswain Tony Barclay of Moelfre Lifeboat Station relates a story about Dwynwen Parry who has been on the crew for many years. She crews on the inshore lifeboat as helm and on the all-weather lifeboat as navigator. The story according to Tony goes:

> Dwyn is basically one of the boys but there are times when we are out for any length of time that it becomes slightly more difficult for Dwyn to go to the loo than the boys. We were out on a shout one night, it was blowing quite hard and we found our casualty just over half way to the Isle of Man. The Port St Mary boat had also been called out and it had been decided that they would tow the casualty back to Port St Mary due to the wind and sea conditions. I decided to stand by while they made a tow fast and while we were hove to, Dwyn decided it would be a good time to try and go to the loo. Well she never told me she was going, I was at the upper steering position and due to the bad weather the cabin door was shut. Apparently Dwyn had just struggled out of her gear and positioned herself on the loo, which is in the fore cabin on the Tyne, when I decided I wanted to re-position round the other side. Down went the throttles and off we went with poor Dwyn holding on for dear life down in the fore cabin.

There is something about a woman's look, you just know you have done something wrong, even in the dark!

Dwyn agrees that Tony has told the tale accurately, but adds:

I had only been a crew member for a few weeks at this time and one of the first to arrive but as the wind was so strong and the waves were rather on the large side (!) I asked Anthony if he preferred to take more experienced crew out with him and I would stand down … his reply was, 'This is the best way for you to see if you can handle it – it's make or break time'. On that note I jumped into my gear and on the boat.

An hour earlier, we had only just finished our training night when a few of us went down to the pub and I had just drunk my first PINT of diet coke(!) when we were alerted. Need I say more? After two hours of swaying and being thrown from one side of the boat to the other we arrived at our casualty. Believe me I have no shame and I was willing to go out on deck like the boys but one of the men suggested I went to the fore cabin while the boat was still. I had to undo my protective gear and my jeans and then with a sigh of relief I offloaded my diet coke! When Tony throttled hard ahead, I was forgotten and with nothing to hold on to, I ended up in a heap on the deck with all my gear around my ankles and much wetter!

Everyone laughed and so did I. It has been a standing joke for the past ten years but Tony was right, it did make me a much stronger person and it certainly made me feel like one of the boys. I now kindly say; 'Right you lot, I'm off to the loo,' and hang off the back end. I know it's not very ladylike but it works much better than my first attempt, and I always do it before we start towing!

Nicki Wood from Sheerness has had to work out her own solution to the toilet issue:

When the bombs went off in London in July 2007, Sheerness lifeboat was tasked to act as a safety boat when Canary Wharf was being evacuated. We left Sheerness and steamed towards London and it took quite a long time to get there. Needless to say when we arrived I needed a wee. We had moored to a buoy on the Thames at Canary Wharf when I decided to go below and 'use the bucket'. When I returned to the deck to throw the wee overboard I noticed a helicopter flying over the boat. I discharged the contents of the bucket in the Thames when my mobile phone rang. It was my husband telling me we were 'live on Sky News'. The incident was very embarrassing to say the least! At least the viewers didn't know what was in the bucket! I now have my own bucket on the ALB. Not even the mechanic will go near it!

Karolyn Rath from Clogher Head says she is always first off the boat at the end of a shout but has to tolerate the men ever asking her 'have you not gone yet?'

Women on the River Thames

When fifty-one people drowned in the River Thames on the night of 20 August 1989 in a collision between the pleasure boat *Marchioness* and the tug *Bowbelle*, there was a formal enquiry into river safety. One of the recommendations from this was for a single agency to have overall responsibility for safety on the River Thames. The outcome was that the Maritime Coastguard Agency made a request to the RNLI to establish a coordinated search and rescue service on the tidal river. The RNLI readily agreed, but knew that although it had an immense amount of relevant experience, this new service would present many unique challenges.

Firstly, the conditions on the River Thames: a six-knot tide, cold water, debris, powerful undercurrents and lots of traffic – over 100,000 people use the river every day and there were on average 100 incidents a year. An immediate requirement was to identify the right sort of boat, as those in the existing fleet were not designed to meet these conditions. Powerful water jet-propelled boats were selected, as these would best cope with the flotsam and jetsam in the river and achieve the required speed to aid the casualty.

To meet the MCA operational requirement for 95 per cent of casualties to be reached within fifteen minutes between the Thames Barrier and Teddington, three permanently manned stations would be established at Gravesend, Tower Pier and Chiswick Pier, and a fourth with a volunteer crew at Teddington. The RNLI had only one permanently manned lifeboat station – at Spurn Head – so to achieve permanent twenty-four-hour cover for three lifeboat stations in metropolitan locations would be a major departure from traditional practice.

The three appointed station managers had a major recruitment task and, from the very beginning, would be seeking women candidates. This lifeboat service would therefore start very differently from the coast, where women joined the crews many years after most of the lifeboat stations were established.

As was predicted when the Thames stations opened on 2 January 2002, they were immediately busy and quickly became the busiest stations in the RNLI. Since then, the Thames lifeboats have had 5,519 call outs and have saved the lives of 346 people (up until the end of 2009). Half their call outs are in hours of darkness, making the difficult river conditions even more challenging. Often the crew rely on a small break of light or a reflection to help them spot a person in the dark, muddy water. They are straining their eyes to see something – maybe just the top of a head, a hand, floating hair or a piece of clothing. Speed of response is critical, and so the demands on the helm are considerable. They must have an accurate knowledge of the river and its tides and bends, but also be alert for the many floating obstructions which could jeopardise a rescue if hit.

Now there are eighteen women on Thames lifeboat crews. Who are they, and what has been their experience serving in this busy service? And, given the significant physical and emotional demands crewing on the Thames places upon them, what does being an RNLI woman mean to them?

Perhaps surprisingly, not all of them live in London. While some commute from the suburbs and home counties, others like Jen Court – full-time helm at Tower Lifeboat Station, and living in Bournemouth – have all established 'home from home' arrangements in order to fulfil the twelve-hour shifts in a four days on, four days off roster. Sue Body lives in London as a medical student at university; home is on Jersey where she is a member of the St Helier lifeboat crew. She was keen to keep up her lifesaving commitment while away from home and the Thames service was the answer.

The reasons why women wanted to become involved with the RNLI on the Thames are as many and varied as on the coast. Both Tanya Houston and Toni Scarr work on the river for the Environment Agency, which has an obvious relevance but does not tell the whole story. Tanya traces her motivation back to her grandfather, whose life had been saved by the RNLI. He then became a keen supporter in Kent, and so Tanya, who loves many water sports, thought this was her way of carrying on her grandfather's work. She successfully persuaded her husband, Sam, to join too. Toni, while working in Jamaica, was shocked that the fishermen there could not swim and it prompted her to think about lifesaving more carefully. Kathy Batts, a self-employed first-aid trainer, also drew on her early experiences of spending time with her father, who was a tug skipper on the Thames – she grew to love the river as much as he. With no boating experience but childhood memories of lifeboat stations in Wales and Cornwall, Laura Ashman, a freelance photographer, was persuaded by the Fowey lifeboat crew to give it a go. Paula Bancroft, a paramedic, read in her employer's house magazine that colleagues were involved and decided to try some 'taster shifts', and Jen Court also started through her work. Her administration job in the RNLI training department at Poole gave her the desire to become a trainer and then to join the Tower crew as a volunteer.

Although a daunting prospect for all, particularly those with no previous experience, joining a Thames lifeboat crew has been very positive. Each person has felt welcomed, encouraged and well trained and supported. The question about whether being a woman makes a difference prompts consistent answers: 'I have been treated as an equal and never asked for or been offered easy options' (Kathy Batts); 'I expect to be capable of all the skills of the male crew' (Jen Court); 'I have never been treated differently and worked really hard to avoid failure and to be respected by my fellow crew members' (Laura Ashman); 'No issues – they accepted me as an equal albeit one with less knowledge of the river' (Paula Bancroft).

The reaction of family and friends is mostly supportive. Tanya Houston thinks her grandma is very proud and convinced that she is out saving 'everyone', but she is careful just who she tells, not wanting to be seen to be bragging – more evidence of the genuine modesty among RNLI crews! Sue Body's friends as often as not are keen to get a lift in the boat … as if! Each woman is very certain it is the support of their respective families, who often have to cope with the practical consequences as well as the anxiety about what they do, which makes the whole service possible.

Having fun lies at the heart of making individuals into an effective team, and the women recognise that the banter, good humour and giving back as good as they get is vital. Toni Scarr remarks that she is not really sure how the men feel about sharing a bunkroom with her, and Tanya Houston admits that 'in training, boobs do tend to get in the way, but it all ends up with a bit of a giggle!' Not living in the same community, the twelve-hour shift and the bunking arrangements mark out significant differences between the Thames crews and coastal lifeboat crews. What is the same, though, is the sense of family that develops. Jen Court refers to it as her 'second' family and Paula Bancroft is appreciative of how training courses at Poole have given her access to the wider RNLI family, while Sue Body confirms that the RNLI is family to almost every crew member she knows.

The RNLI lifeboat service on the River Thames is highly effective and efficient, making an immense difference in London for those in danger in or by the water. Women are well represented in the crews and as such reflect the emergency services in the capital in which there are also many women. All the RNLI women share the conviction that mixed crews enhance the service by providing a more balanced support network. They agree that women bring different strengths and offer a different and healthy perspective. Sometimes the public is surprised about women's involvement, but more often than not their presence is taken for granted. Jen Court, who attracted a lot of media attention when she was appointed as full-time helm at Tower Lifeboat Station, worries that such publicity could detract from the fact that 'we all do the same job'.

Many of the shouts on the Thames involve people attempting suicide – the river acts as a magnet for distressed and disturbed people and sadly not all call outs are successful. It is not surprising that the crew has poignant memories of incidents where they were successful in giving a person a 'second chance'. Toni Scarr recalls feeling very humbled when, under Battersea Bridge in very difficult fast moving water, the crew rescued a 'jumper' who later wrote and thanked them. Sue Body successfully resuscitated a person and remembers how wonderful it was to feel the pulse start again. She received letters of thanks from both London Coastguard and the RNLI for this rescue.

Thames crews have their share of funny incidents, too. Kathy Batts laughed when rescuing two men – one rather overweight – and a dog who had fallen from the pontoon at Thurrock Yacht Club. The men were not wearing lifejackets but the dog was! Tanya Houston has not forgotten the last words of a naval officer, who was transferring from the lifeboat to his ship: 'Don't worry, nothing ever happens.' Immediately after these blithe words, he fell in! One of the situations all crew must learn to cope with is the large number of people who sometimes gather to watch a rescue. Jen Court's first shout as helm occurred at 5p.m., when thousands of commuters are on the move – it was nerve-wracking to have so many people watching from the bank.

With specific reasons of their own for doing so, the women of Thames crews are all givers. They readily acknowledge how much, in return, they receive; being a member of a lifeboat crew is life-changing. Laura Ashman summarises what most feel:

> …it helps to put things into perspective for me, with my job you need that. To be real. To meet real people. Also to learn and be challenged. It is great to be able to do something useful once in a while that has the potential to change in a positive way not just my life but someone else's.

The most unexpected incident of all happened to Paula Bancroft, who was completely unaware of what was afoot when she agreed to role-play the casualty in a first-aid exercise. All of Chiswick crew were in on the act and even made her check the boat camera so that everything was recorded. Lying 'unconscious' in the lifeboat she was roused by a person in full gear, carrying a life ring painted in gold, proposing marriage! 'How could I say no? I would have been in the drink!' laughs Paula. The wedding was on a boat on the Thames and her taxi was a lifeboat. Now they have baby girl, named Beatrix Alice.

Medals for bravery

The RNLI Committee of Management has awarded medals for bravery to a total of twenty-two women. Of these, nineteen were presented in the nineteenth century when there were no women serving on lifeboat crews. The intention in those days was to acknowledge special acts of bravery performed by women – some were in support of a lifeboat rescue, and some were not. Apart from Grace Darling's rescue, which has been widely documented and publicised, there is no detailed information for the other medallists. What little there is has been extracted from the RNLI Committee of Management minutes by Barry Cox, RNLI Honorary Librarian.

1838 – Grace Darling

7 September 1838 – early in the morning, while on watch at the Longstone Lighthouse, where her father was Keeper, Grace saw the ship SS *Forfarshire* strike Big Harcar rock and break in two. She reported this to her father William, and with a telescope they kept watch on the ship. When morning light came they saw survivors. With trepidation, William agreed that his daughter, who was just twenty-three years old, should join him in their small open boat, a coble, to row to their rescue. He knew they could reach the wreck, but because the return would be against the tide and the storm, he would need the help of some of the survivors.

After rowing hard through huge waves for about a mile, they found eight men and one woman alive and clinging on to the rocks. William jumped out of the boat, leaving Grace to hold the boat steady with the oars in the sea in readiness for taking the survivors on board. This was a tremendous feat of boat handling skill for anyone, let alone a diminutive young woman. William helped five people into the boat: a woman who was found holding her two dead children in her arms, and four men, one with a broken leg. With the help of two of the men, William and Grace rowed back to the Lighthouse where Mrs Darling, helped by Grace, cared for them all. William and two of the stronger survivors rowed back to the wreck to complete the rescue.

News of this rescue spread rapidly throughout the country. The fact that a young woman had shown such courage captured the imagination of the public. In no time she became a 'Victorian Heroine' in the full glare of the press and the public. Newspapers were quick to scoop stories about Grace and her family; artists begged for her to sit for portraits – she sat for seven portraits in twelve days! William Wordsworth, the Poet Laureate, wrote a poem, special boat trips were organised as people flocked to Longstone Lighthouse to see her, and Grace Darling souvenirs appeared for sale – for entrepreneurs this became a lucrative 'industry'.

Grace was deluged with congratulatory letters and gifts, but also with requests – for locks of her hair, for advice, for money. It was completely overwhelming for a young person who had lived a sheltered life. Help came from the Duke of Northumberland, who stepped in to act as her advisor and guardian. Grace hated all the attention, holding firmly to her view that she had done nothing outstanding. She developed a cough and, believing that she needed a rest, her parents organised for her to stay with friends at Wooler. In fact she had tuberculosis, and as her condition worsened her longing to be home grew stronger. Her sister, who lived at Bamburgh, took her home, and there she died on 20 October 1842, just twenty-six years old. Many thought that her life had been shortened by the pressures of so much attention. She was buried in St Aidan's Churchyard in Bamburgh, opposite the cottage where she was born.

A museum housing a collection of Grace Darling memorabilia and telling the story of her courageous rescue was opened in Bamburgh in 1938. It had many visitors, but became increasingly in need of refurbishment. The joint efforts of local volunteers and the RNLI Heritage Trust secured funding to extend and modernise the museum, which reopened in 2008.

Grace and her father were awarded the Gold Medal of the Royal Humane Society and the RNLI Silver Medal.

All female recipients of the RNLI Silver Medal
1847 – Misses Margaret and Martha Llewellyn
22 October 1846 – in severe weather, a smack, the *Margaret* of Barmouth, became stranded on the beach at Fishguard. The two sisters waded into the surf to assist a couple of men to rescue three seamen.

1847 – Mrs Georgia Vilhelmina Fisher
March 1847 – when the British ship *Marwood* was wrecked on the Faroe Islands the crew attempted to scramble ashore over rocks. They became swamped in the surf and one of the men was so battered that he appeared to be dead. Several islanders came to their rescue but only one, a clergyman's wife, understood resuscitation, and after much persistence was successful in reviving him.

1856 – Misses Grace Tait and Ellen Petrie
23 May 1856 – a small fishing boat capsized in Blumull Sound, which lies between the Shetland Islands of Unst and Yell. In severe weather, the women joined Miss Tait's father to row to the boat, where they were able to save the lives of two of the four fishermen. This was achieved at great risk to themselves, in a racing tide in one of the most dangerous sounds in the Shetlands. Each received two pounds.

1858 – Mrs May Stout Hectorson Moar
9 September 1858 – seeing that a boat with four men on board had capsized off Burra Ness in the Shetland Islands, she attached a rope to herself and descended a cliff to a point where she could throw the rope and a lifebuoy to two of the men. With the aid of two women holding the rope fast at the top of the cliff, she then drew them through the surf to the shore. The other two men were rescued by Mr Moar, for which he was awarded ten shillings.

1864 – Miss Alice Bell Le Geyt
4 August 1864 – while on holiday in Lyme Regis she saw two boys fall into the sea from the outer pier. As she was in a pleasure boat with a lady friend, she rowed through the surf to save them.

1871 – Miss Jane Campbell

27 September 1871 – seeing a man floating in the sea in a very exhausted state, she rushed into the heavy surf and resuscitated him. This was off the Drogheda Bar on the River Boyne, County Louth. The sailor had been on the ship *Manly*, which had become wrecked in a strong easterly gale.

1879 – Misses Ellen Frances, Gertrude Rose, Mary Katherine and Beatrice May Prideaux Brune, and Miss Nora O'Shaughnessy

2 October 1879 – five young women were enjoying their relaxing trip in a rowing boat, which was being towed by the assistant coxswain of Padstow in his fishing boat. When a sudden squall blew up, their attention was drawn to a capsized boat and people in the water. Immediately they asked to be cast off in order to row to the casualties to give help. Anxious for their safety the assistant coxswain tried to dissuade them, but they were determined and set off 'rowing like tigers' through the heavy surf. They saved one man from drowning and with great difficulty got him into their boat.

1884 – Mrs Whyte

28 October 1884 – in a heavy gale the Dundee steamer *William Hope* foundered in Aberdour Bay, Fife. Mrs Whyte went to a place on the beach where she was able to catch hold of a rope thrown to her by one of the crew and wound it around her body. By anchoring her feet firmly on the beach, six men were able to reach safety.

1887 – Misses Maria and Josephine Horsford

3 November 1887 – rowing a very small boat, the sisters went with William Sullivan to the rescue of four people who had been in a sailing boat which had capsized in Courtmacsherry Bay, County Cork.

1888 – Mrs Wallace and Miss Ellen Blyth

12 April 1888 – four men stranded on the ship *Burns and Bessie* were rescued by the Assistant Keeper of the Point of Ayr Lighthouse, William Wallace and a temporary assistant, TA Christian. Helping with the lines to bring the men ashore was his wife and the Head Keeper's daughter.

2004 – the first woman crew member to be awarded a medal for gallantry

Over 116 years were to pass before the next woman received a bravery award from the RNLI. In radically different circumstances from Victorian days, the awardee in 2004 was not only a lifeboat crew member, she was also the helm.

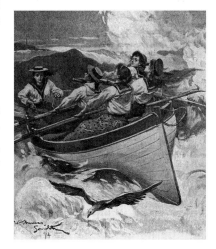

The four Prideaux Brune sisters and Nora O'Shaughnessy rowing 'like tigers'.

Aileen Jones, Porthcawl

The RNLI press release describes the rescue thus:

24 August 2004

Jones, the helmsman of the RNLI Porthcawl lifeboat, braved gale force winds, rough seas and a three metre swell to rescue a fishing vessel, Gower Pride, which suffered engine failure. The skipper and an injured fisherman were on board. The entire crew of the Porthcawl lifeboat faced atrocious sea conditions and twice managed to attach a towline – the second time by putting Crewman Emms on board the fishing vessel after the first towline broke. At that moment the Gower Pride was hit by a large breaking wave on the starboard side and was thrown against the lifeboat. Helmsman Jones quickly manoeuvred the vessels apart, and continued – with great skill – to use the inshore lifeboat to keep the rolling fishing vessel away from danger. They began a slow tow against high seas, which at times lifted the bow of the lifeboat precariously out of the water.

By this time the Mumbles all-weather lifeboat had been called to assist and the crews were able to transfer the tow from the smaller Porthcawl lifeboat. The two lifeboats were able then to complete the perilous journey home and get the skipper and his injured crewman to safety.

What can Aileen add to this factual account? She recalls being fascinated by the sea on the morning of 24 August – it was so extraordinarily rough. There had been plans to go for a day out to Ilfracombe on the *Balmoral*, but the sailing was cancelled. She first heard about the fishing boat in trouble on the VHF radio and went straight to the lifeboat station. She was the first helm to arrive and as is the practice at the station, she took command. She made a decision about the approach to the casualty, realising she would need to take a different line from normal because of the size of the waves. As it was, they bounced off every one, at times the lifeboat standing on end. Her thoughts focused on how she was going to get the *Gower Pride* back. She recalls her concern when fellow crewman Mark Burtonwood was knocked down, but then once the Mumbles lifeboat joined them, her total concentration was on the slow tow home, keeping the boat stable and away from the banks. Back on shore, she thought it a job well done, but essentially an ordinary shout. Such is the modesty of a woman who from childhood wanted to be on the lifeboat.

As a teenager, Aileen recalls spending as much time as she could at the station, offering to be helpful but now suspecting that she was probably a 'pain in the neck'. On reaching seventeen, she filled in the application form but was turned down: 'I was given different excuses, but it didn't put me off – it was in my blood.' The only route in was by forcing her husband to be, Stephen, to become interested in the lifeboat. Happily he joined the crew and this gave his wife Aileen a legitimate way in as a helper. Eventually in 1995 she was accepted on to the crew and immediately loved every minute of it. There was no problem in bringing her two children, Daniel and Frances, to the station, so that enabled Aileen to be fully involved. Something significant must have rubbed off on them, because both joined the crew when they were old enough.

The RNLI was keen to publicise the first award of a medal to a woman for 116 years and so Aileen had something of a 'Grace Darling experience'. She works as a nursery assistant and had to get a day off work for the press call. From RNLI HQ came a press expert to help her, but Aileen remembers feeling so overawed by the barrage of instructions of what to do and what not to do, that she went for a walk to calm down. In retrospect, having had no previous press exposure, she realises that she was something of 'a lamb to the slaughter'. Thankfully most of the press were pleasant and helpful. On the day of the awards ceremony in London, Aileen was on the go from 4a.m. with TV and radio interviews and endless photographs: 'they all want the same, do they know how tiring it is?' After the Duke of Kent had presented her medal, everyone in the Barbican Hall gave Aileen a standing ovation. She remembers thinking 'please sit down!' Part of her concern was being the focus of so much attention when she clearly knew that without the other members of the crew that day, she could have achieved nothing. This was compounded by her worry that she as the woman medal winner was drawing attention away from the other crew members who were also receiving much deserved medals that day.

These sensitivities tell so much about Aileen Jones, the woman who says that serving on a lifeboat crew is her way of life. She is adamant that she and her family have received more than she has given: a huge circle of friends, the chance to do good in her community, and the chance to be recognised by them. She sees the lifeboat station community as an extension of her own family, and knows how much they all look out for each other. She takes pleasure in educating the next generation of lifeboat crew and just wishes that every young person could join. Aileen contemplates her retirement from the crew with trepidation: 'Maybe I'll volunteer to drive the tractor, but after the boat it's …' She hesitates, but it's easy to fill in her words. Some of her energy will go to worrying about son Daniel, who she knows has a long career ahead of him on the lifeboat: 'It terrifies me – but I can't say anything.' The words of a courageous woman – one who turned her own back on terror.

2007 – two women awarded medals in one year
Dr Christine Bradshaw, Longhope

Some people have made the decision to join a lifeboat crew after they themselves have been rescued. Christine Bradshaw was once rescued when surfing in Cornwall, but although she was extremely appreciative, it was not that event which finally prompted her to volunteer – it was another much more dramatic experience.

Christine is a doctor who, on 11 November 2006, was working as a relief GP on the island of Hoy in Orkney. The practice provides essential medical support for the Longhope lifeboat when it is launched and there is known to be a serious medical casualty. For her, the day started quite normally in helping the Ladies Lifeboat Guild clear up after the Christmas Bazaar that she had opened the previous day when the knock came on the door. This was the first indication that she was needed, but she had no idea of what a huge task was ahead of her.

Out in the Pentland Firth, the deck of an oil tanker *FR8 Venture* had been swamped by a huge wave, seriously injuring three of the crew. Both the lifeboat and the coastguard helicopter were needed if the men's lives were to be saved, and Christine's expertise would be essential. She picks up the story:

> The mechanic John Budge spoke clearly and calmly to me on the lifeboat and explained that
> I would have to be winched down onto the tanker and advised me that I didn't have to do

it if I didn't want to. At the time the thought of not going did not enter my head. There was only one size survival suit, large and at 5'3" I was swamped in it and trying to work in it on the tanker was incredibly hot and sweaty.

By the time they reached the oil tanker, the swell was fifteen metres and a sudden hailstorm made conditions even more dangerous as Christine prepared to be winched onto the deck of the tanker, which was completely awash:

> Winching off the lifeboat was a struggle due to the rise and fall of the boat. I was crouching on the deck, hanging on against the rise and fall in the swell whilst the winchman was trying to get on board.

Eventually, thanks to the great skill of both the lifeboat and helicopter crews, Christine was safely winched onto the tanker deck. She found one crewman already dead, one on the very brink of death who did not respond to her endeavours to resuscitate and one who had serious spinal injuries that required stabilisation:

> I felt enormous sympathy for the crew and what they had just been through. They had done their best, as had I, and after the failed resuscitation they could not believe their crewmates were dead; one of the deceased had four children.

The next task was to airlift the injured man so that he could be flown to hospital. The towering waves made this very difficult, but it was skilfully achieved. The helicopter winchman told Christine that these were the worst conditions he had ever been winched in. Having seen her patient safely into Aberdeen Hospital, Christine now needed to get back to Hoy – she was still in her oversized survival suit, with all her medical kit, but with no phone and no money. Fortunately the lifeboat crew persuaded the helicopter team to drop her back to Hoy as, without her, the island had no doctor. She was landed in a muddy field, where the wellie-like shoes of her survival suit got stuck in the mud and suddenly Christine realised how tired she felt.

She was disappointed not to meet up with the lifeboat crew immediately, but they were recovering the two dead bodies from the tanker. When the crew returned Christine saw they were subdued – it had been a tough day for everyone. She was still on duty so she went home, quietly wishing she could turn off her bleeper. She then had a difficult night:

> I couldn't sleep with everything running through my mind – what if … in terms of my medical treatment, could I have saved the second crewman if I'd have done something differently, etc. There were visions of the previous day in my mind.

Christine was surprised to receive a medal for what she considered to be a normal part of her duty as a doctor, but she felt great pride that her efforts were to be recognised in this way – as did her family. She agreed to participate in all the media activity in order that the RNLI might benefit. It was time-consuming and demanding, but such is her admiration for the work of the RNLI she wanted to do all she could to raise awareness. She enjoyed

Dr Christine Bradshaw of Longhope, awarded the RNLI
Silver Medal for bravery.

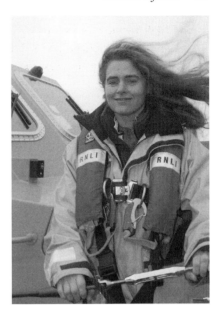

appearing alongside Sophie Grant-Crookston
(see page 59) and says of her: 'She is a legend, a
real gem, unassuming, very kind and a very strong
swimmer – she well deserved her medal.' Sophie
gives an almost identical description of Christine!

Having considered it once before, the tanker
rescue was the ultimate prompt for Christine to
join a lifeboat crew – Longhope. Here she was
held in the highest esteem and warmly welcomed.
For Christine it is an obvious extension of her
professional commitment to saving life, but there
is more:

> I enjoy the camaraderie of the crew, the banter and
> the fun we all have which far outweighs the unpleasant cold dark nights out training in the
> winter, when we would all rather be doing something else. Being a female crew member
> makes me feel proud to be female as a demonstration that women can do it as well as the men,
> as long as it is done as well as the men.

Future crew

Grace Wadsworth

When the Winter 2009 issue of *the Lifeboat* dropped through the letterbox of RNLI supporters, a smiling face greeted them from the cover – Grace Wadsworth from Lyme Regis.
She was chosen as the image to lead an article about a new scheme to attract young recruits
to lifeboating and lifeguarding.

Grace, who is currently at school studying for A-levels, became involved initially at Lyme
Regis Lifeboat Station to complete the service section for her Duke of Edinburgh Award.
Her father, Tim, is a member of the crew there and as Grace is a keen sailor, it seemed a
good choice and she also had the company of two other young people doing their Duke of
Edinburgh Award. At first they were treated as shore crew, helping out with the launch and
recovery of the lifeboat and they were given a pager so that they could have the experience
and the excitement of attending a shout. For Grace, it was a very positive experience, and
by the time she had completed her gold award the lifeboat service had become a big part
of her life. She had experienced 'the feeling of pride you get from being in the organisation
and saving other people's lives', and wanted more.

Now she is training as a full crew member and it is a 'first' for Lyme Regis Lifeboat
Station, which has not had a woman on the crew before. Grace says that her approach has
been 'to get stuck into things and show people that I wasn't any different and that I could
do things just as good as them – and sometimes better!' Occasionally she is at the receiving

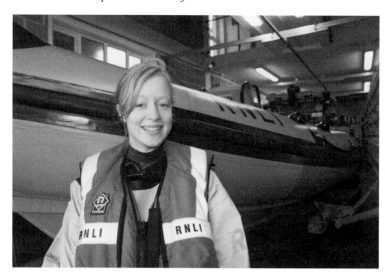

Grace Wadsworth – a young member of Lyme Regis lifeboat crew.

end of what she sees as a sexist remark, such as 'are you sure that's not too heavy for you?' Grace realises that it is nothing very serious and it is a new experience for the crew and hopes that she will pave the way for other women to become involved at Lyme Regis – she thinks it is about time they did!

She has a busy life combining her studies with a part-time job and a range of interests. For her, being on a lifeboat crew is something different from normal teenager activities and has given her the opportunity to meet many new people. The training has given her a lot of new skills, and one she especially values is the ability to think more clearly in emergency situations.

Grace plans to go to university to read History, which will mean a break in crewing, but she aims to be back as soon as possible – for 'the pride and the buzz you get in helping to save a person's life'.

What would Sir William Hillary say if he were to walk into an RNLI boathouse today and find women on the crew – women like Emily Bettison at his own lifeboat station in Douglas? He was unquestionably a forward-thinking person, so one has to think that he would welcome the tremendous energy, commitment and skill that women are bringing to the service. It is hard to be certain – he might share some of the preconceptions about the capabilities of women that are still held by people who look askance when told that women serve on today's lifeboat crews. His own – often quoted – words were: 'With courage, everything is possible.' He proved it, and so have these women. May there be many more who do …

three

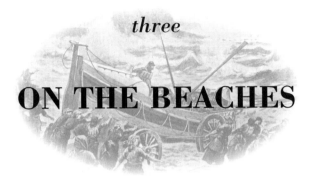

ON THE BEACHES

'Oh I do love to be beside the seaside …' Words from an old music hall song that many of us would agree with! Usually a day on the beach is a happy experience and we take home good memories of the sea. Sometimes, though, things can go wrong, often very quickly. When someone drowns, the memories of a day at the seaside are of a tragedy.

Could the RNLI do anything to help save lives on our beaches? This question was prompted by the statistic that on average 400 people drown off our beaches every year. With much relevant experience in saving life at sea, it was very possible that the RNLI could make a difference on our beaches, but it was a proposition that needed to be pursued carefully. In the summer of 2001, trial beach lifeguard services were set up on twenty-two beaches in Cornwall and Dorset. At the end of the season an evaluation was made to determine whether the RNLI would develop and expand the service.

Establishing a brand new service within a well-established organisation brings a number of challenges, and from the outset it was clear that some aspects of the RNLI would be transferable, but some would not. Providing good quality equipment and thorough training would be as essential for beach lifeguarding as for lifeboating, so this was implemented immediately. Exclusive use of volunteers to run the service would not be a realistic option. On a beach, seconds really count and can make the difference between saving a life or not. Beaches must be continually manned during daylight hours, and that meant engaging large numbers of lifeguards. As it was to be a seasonal service, the plan was to have predominantly paid lifeguards supported by a network of volunteers for weekends and other peak times.

That first trial was a great success with the lifeguard service immediately proving its worth, and since then it has been progressively expanded. Importantly, it is now an integral part of the RNLI enabling the organisation to provide a coordinated rescue service from the beach to the open sea. Many individuals and families have good reason to be grateful for the help they have received from RNLI lifeguards – for some it was simply a plaster placed on a cut and for others it was advice on where to swim safely. For some fortunate people, it was to be saved from death by drowning.

Now the scale of the operation is huge. In 2009, RNLI lifeguards attended 9,536 incidents and assisted 11,027 people. They will be on 152 beaches in 2010 and there are plans to double the number in the next three years. They believe that 95 per cent of their work

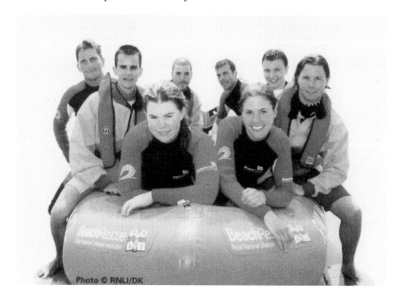

Photo © RNLI/DK

The first RNLI
lifeguards on
Sandbanks Beach,
Dorset.

is preventative. On the beaches, in schools and local communities they offer beach safety advice in a friendly and positive way with the aim of preventing an accident before it happens.

'Women lifeguards? I've never heard anyone say we should not be part of it'

Setting up a new service in the twenty-first century meant that from the outset, women were welcomed as lifeguards. In the first trials there were just four women. The number has grown significantly since then, partly reflecting the growth of the service but also a change of emphasis in recruitment. In 2008 a soft approach was used to attract more women into lifeguard roles by using more female imagery in recruitment material. It was effective; the number of women doubled between 2007 and 2008. In 2009, there were 744 lifeguards, of which 145 were female. The majority of women lifeguards are aged between eighteen and twenty-four years – a younger age profile than for lifeboat crew.

The RNLI lifeguard service operates on designated beaches between May and September, and so most paid lifeguards find alternative employment during the winter months. Many of them follow the sun and go to the southern hemisphere to lifeguard. There is a small permanent team of managers and supervisors who work throughout the year to support and develop the service, and two of them are women.

Kelly Blackburn, East Lindsey

Kelly was no stranger to the RNLI when she applied for the post of Area Lifeguard Supervisor for East Lindsey. She is a member of the Cleethorpes lifeboat crew and has been since 2004. A very committed one too – she won a special award in 2008 for being the RNLI student who achieved the best results on the Ocean Training RYA theory distance learning course. Kelly is currently the Station Training Coordinator at Cleethorpes and a prospective helm. A keen competitive swimmer at school, Kelly qualified as a pool and beach lifeguard, which led her into employment as a Beach Safety Officer with the local council.

By 2007 she realised two things: firstly, she was ready to move on to another job; and secondly, it was the RNLI she wanted to work for. What, though, might be available for a woman who definitely did not want to work indoors? Months of searching the recruitment website was rewarded when the Lifeguard Supervisor post was advertised. Now she has responsibility for three beaches on the Lincolnshire coast – the first woman ever to be appointed to this position.

Good teamwork is what Kelly firmly believes will underpin the success of the service she is responsible for. Throughout her working life she has always been in teams where she was one of a few women, or the youngest – or both! Her policy, especially in challenging situations, has been complete honesty with everyone and certainly with herself:

> Successful teams are those where everyone has a common goal and where everyone knows each other's capabilities and trusts each other. I tell my lifeguard teams to play to their strengths – everyone has proven they are capable and can do all aspects of the job. But everyone has preferences and if the time and situation allow then they can put the best person forward for the job at hand.

Developing her team of young and newly qualified lifeguards is a key responsibility in this role, and it means a lot to Kelly when she sees them apply their training to real life scenarios which they have mostly never faced before. She particularly recalls an incident when two of her team went to see if they could assist coastguards and paramedics with a casualty evacuation from the beach. As it happened they were not really needed, but they chose to stay – just in case. By doing so, they witnessed the prolonged resuscitation of a man who had collapsed. After forty-five minutes of CPR (Cardiac Pulmonary Resuscitation) and several shocks from a defibrillator, he started to breathe again. This was a happy ending, but a rare one, given the length of time he had not been breathing. For the two lifeguards it was a profound experience early in their career, and one which Kelly is convinced helped them to understand their responsibilities as a lifeguard.

Not all incidents end so happily, though, as Kelly knows only too well. Her experience of seeing how people's fortunes change so quickly and with no warning has made her much more philosophical. She worries less about trivialities and seeks out something positive that can be learnt from every incident. Working on the beaches, she is constantly striving with her team to make sure that their experience of a visit to the seaside is pleasurable and safe. Saving life? Kelly answers with typical modesty, 'naturally it is a great feeling'.

Elin Jones, Ceredigion

The challenge of setting up a new RNLI lifeguard service along part of the Ceredigion coast was what first attracted Elin to the job. She had not previously worked with the RNLI, but did have lots of experience beach lifeguarding along this coastline as a swimming teacher, lifeguard assessor and staff trainer with the local council. Surf Lifesaving is a passion for Elin, her husband and two daughters. They are all involved with the Surf

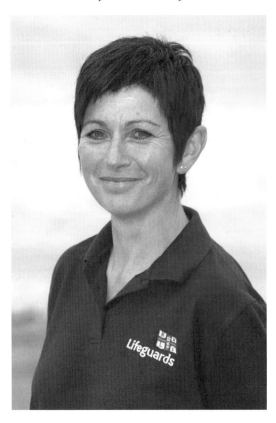

Elin Jones, RNLI Lifeguard Supervisor, Ceredigion.

Lifesaving Club at Newport Sands, where Elin trains everyone, from the 'Nippers' to those who take the Beach Lifeguard Award.

She said goodbye to her proud and supportive family and friends when, having been offered the post, she was required to attend a supervisor course at the Lifeboat College in Poole. Elin did not know what to expect and was surprised to find that she was the only woman on her course of ten people. Immediately she knew she was in for a big challenge! And so it was – both physically and mentally – and the memory of the experience will stay with her forever. Looking back, she recalls how the team spirit was built up during the week and she made some very good friends – people who will remain so throughout her RNLI career. It was only at the end of the week that one of the trainers told her that the experience could have gone one of two ways:'either the men would chew me up and spit me out, or embrace my company and what I had to offer.' Elin's determination made sure it was the latter.

Back on her patch, Elin works with seven male colleagues who treat her no differently, and nor would she want them to. She does feel that on occasion she has to work harder to prove herself, but knows this is very typical of her approach to life. She puts her faith in good teamwork and has committed herself and members of her team to a challenge as part of the team-building process. They are entered into a quadrathon (swimming, kayaking, cycling, running). 'I decided on this event as it would be a great challenge for the team. We need lots of team training so I've put a training plan in place and I don't know whether they'll hate me or love me at the end of it!'

Elin's family is still behind her though. Her elder daughter Megan completed her first session with the RNLI lifeguards in Pembokeshire last summer and has signed up for the next. Little sister Molly – who's not so little, taller than her sister in fact – can't wait to become a beach lifeguard. Molly continues to train and compete for the Club and spends her summers on the beach.

Medal for gallantry awarded to RNLI lifeguard

Sophie Grant-Crookston, Carrick
'She did it without a thought for her own safety.'

Sophie grew up near Newquay in Cornwall, where she and her family loved to spend as much time as they could on the beach. Her parents were keen for her to be involved with the local surf lifesaving activities, believing that she would be safer in the water if she had trained properly. Sophie learnt quickly and started competing at an early age. Later, as is the custom in surfing clubs, she became involved in the voluntary beach patrols with the lifeguards. When the RNLI took over the service in Carrick in 2001, she signed up and has been an RNLI lifeguard there for nine seasons. As lifeguarding is seasonal, she has other jobs too, such as nanny to four little girls and swim coaching.

Sophie welcomed the immediate difference made by the RNLI. There was better equipment, and more of it, for the lifeguards to use – so important because her part of Cornwall has very popular surfing beaches that get crowded with tourists of the bucket and spade variety. She has mainly worked on Perranporth and Holywell Bay beaches where there is a potent mix of dangerous natural elements, including surf, rip tides, rocks and large numbers of people – many of them lacking in knowledge of how to stay safe in these conditions. The lifeguards are kept very busy at Perranporth and although Sophie loves it that way, she says that there are times when you don't get time to breathe. In these conditions they get pushed to their limit and often experience great adrenaline rushes. This is when the value of a strong team spirit becomes very clear, as when the lifeguards had to organise a mass rescue of 100 people on Perranporth Beach – happily with no fatalities.

It was a single surfer in trouble near Perranporth that triggered a dramatic rescue by the RNLI lifeguard team. Sophie's contribution was so outstanding that she was awarded the RNLI Bronze Meal for Gallantry. The incident, in which Sophie certainly risked her life, took place on 22 September 2006.

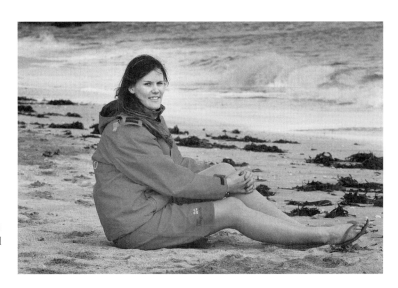

Sophie
Grant-Crookston of
Carrick, awarded the
RNLI Bronze Medal
for gallantry in 2007.
(Mike Thomas)

In powerful two-metre waves, a surfer lost his board and was forced to take refuge on a narrow rock shelf. It was a very dangerous place to be; the waves were crashing over the rocks and with the tide rising fast, it would not be long before the whole ledge was submerged. With difficulty the surfer clung on, but he got cut and bruised as his body thumped against the rocks. Fortunately someone had seen his plight and contacted the duty lifeguards. Sophie was one of them, and the others were David Green, Kris O'Neill and Robin Howell. Together they assessed the situation and decided that the sea was too rough to take their Rescue Water Craft right up to the rocks. They agreed a plan for two of them to take it as close as possible and then for one of them to swim to rescue the surfer.

Sophie volunteered, and remembers the strength of the sea as she swam through the waves that were taking her in every direction but the one she wanted to go in. She had to swim through thirty metres of raging sea. When she got to the rock ledge it was difficult to climb on to it. To make it easier she took her swim fins off, but while she was giving her attention to this manoeuvre a wave swept her away and she had to put them back on again. After a great struggle she heaved herself onto the rock where the surfer was waiting, exhausted, injured and in shock. She attached a rescue tube to him and spoke encouragingly to him until Robin and David arrived in an Inshore Rescue Boat. As the waves were so powerful, they had to judge the optimum moment to make an approach. Sophie had to make a judgement too – just when she and the surfer should re-enter the water. When a lull in the waves eventually came, the IRB was skilfully manoeuvred into place and Sophie and the surfer jumped into the water and she helped him swim back to the boat. Safely back on the beach, the surfer was given oxygen and both his and Sophie's cuts were treated.

The teamwork of David, Kris, Robin and Sophie was quite exceptional and, as is very typical of RNLI lifesavers, each of them unselfishly gives most credit to the others. Sophie, knowing how big a rescue she had been involved in, quickly told her father, who was very proud of her achievement. Her great sadness is that he died soon after so never got to know that she had been awarded a medal for her bravery.

Sophie was the first woman RNLI lifeguard to receive a bravery medal and says that although she is immensely proud, she can hardly believe it. Her real hope is that it might encourage more women to get involved in the service. The medal was presented to her by HRH the Duke of Kent at the 2007 Awards Ceremony. There she met Dr Christine Bradshaw who was receiving her medal. They were thrown together by circumstance but easily struck up a very warm friendship. Sophie well remembers being amazed and daunted by the media attention and was grateful that she and Christine faced it together. Masses of TV and radio interviews at the time of the ceremony were followed by an invitation to appear on a TV programme, Ben Fogle's *Extreme Dreams*.

Sophie has come to look back on this as a very positive experience. Now she is confident and happy to appear in front of TV cameras to speak about RNLI lifeguards. In the back of her mind she carries the thought that it may just make people aware of the contribution made by women to the RNLI. Without question, she is a woman who carries her courage and her achievements with exceptional modesty.

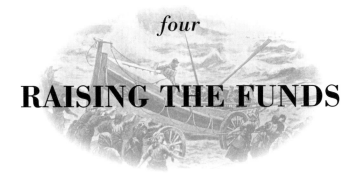

four

RAISING THE FUNDS

Some people are amazed that the RNLI receives no state funding to run the lifeboat service. Those who are closely involved with the organisation relish its financial independence and argue that this freedom from Government involvement lies at the heart of such a magnificent record of achievement in saving lives. There is a powerful and effective chemistry in volunteer fundraisers supporting volunteer lifesavers. Sir William Hillary, the founder of the RNLI, anticipated this when in 1824 he was campaigning to establish a national lifeboat service:

> Who is there, to whom such an Institution, once became known, that would refuse his aid? It is a cause which extends from the palace to the cottage, in which politics and party cannot have any share, and which addresses itself with equal force to all the best feelings of every class of the state.

Would he then have anticipated that the best allies of this cause would be women? It seems unlikely, but thanks in part to thousands of generous, resourceful and innovative women the RNLI has received the money it needed to establish and develop a world-class lifesaving service.

Ladies' Lifeboat Auxiliary Committees – the first women fundraisers

Early financial support for the newly founded RNLI came from individual subscriptions and donations. Archives of old ledgers listing each and every contribution, beautifully penned in copperplate handwriting, bear testimony to the generosity of many individuals minded to help the new service. Money flowing in confirmed Sir William Hillary's confidence that people would give.

Such a happy state of financial affairs – while sufficient to facilitate his aims to expand the service, improve the design and build of lifeboats and provide pensions for the families of crew for a number of years – was not to last. In fact, scrutiny of the accounts in 1890 would show that a high proportion of the Institution's income had been contributed by just 100 people, and they had bequeathed money specifically to build lifeboats. In that year, when the population of the United Kingdom was 37.7 million, just 25,000 people had made a donation to the RNLI – much more palace than cottage!

It was a disaster in 1886 off the coast of Lancashire, the like of which had not been experienced by the RNLI in its sixty-two-year history, which started a sequence of initiatives. These eventually positioned women at the very heart of fundraising on the scale that was required to ensure the regular flow of income needed to sustain a consistent and reliable lifeboat service.

In a severe gale on a December night, a German ship – *Mexico* – sailing from Liverpool to Guayaquil in South America encountered difficulties and was swept into the Ribble Estuary. Knowing that the ship and its twelve crew members were in dire danger, the Captain ordered the firing of distress signals. Three lifeboats responded: St Anne's, Southport and Lytham. The tragedy of the night is that two of those lifeboats capsized as they struggled with the raging sea and twenty-seven men were drowned. Only Lytham lifeboat returned intact, having successfully rescued all the crew from the *Mexico*.

Such a great loss for the families and their communities was appalling. Public expressions of concern for the families of the dead crewmen were fuelled by the media. The attention of the Poet Laureate, Clement Scott, was aroused, and he wrote a poem, 'The Warriors of the Sea', drawing attention to the suffering and the bravery of the women who could only watch and hope:

> … Along the sands of Southport, brave women held their breath,
> For they knew that those who loved them were fighting hard with death.
> A cheer went out from Lytham! The tempest toss'd it back,
> As the gallant lads of Lancashire bent to the waves attack;
> And girls who dwell about St Anne's, with faces white with fright,
> Pray'd God would still the tempest, that dark December night.
> Sons, husbands, brothers, lovers, they'd given up their all,
> These noble English women, heart sick at duty's call;
> But not a cheer, or tear or prayer, from those who bent the knee,
> Came out across the waves to nerve those Warriors of the sea! …

Help for the dependents was urgently needed, and thanks to Lord Derby and Charles Macara, a Manchester businessman who lived at St Anne's-on-the-Sea, a disaster fund was launched. Money flowed in from individuals and from a special appeal by *The Daily Telegraph*. However, Charles Macara had serious concerns about this approach to fundraising, which successfully brought in money when the public heartstrings were touched by a tragedy, but not on a predictable or long-term basis. His business head told him that to better balance RNLI income with its expenditure, the sensible thing would be to approach broader constituencies of support. In his own words, 'Bring the charity into the streets and the streets into the charity'.

He organised the first ever Lifeboat Saturday – it took place on 17 October 1891 in Manchester – and amazingly raised £5,500. It is the stuff of RNLI legend, because it acted

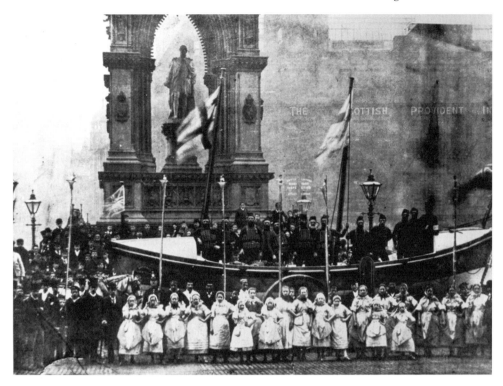

The first Lifeboat Saturday held in Manchester on 17 October 1891.

as a model to be replicated all over the country for almost 120 years, bringing in many thousands of pounds while raising public awareness of the work of lifeboat crews.

Supporting Charles Macara in his work to improve RNLI finances was his wife Marion, who knew first hand of the agonies of waiting for the safe return of a lifeboat crew. She had already conscripted a group of ladies to assist in collecting money on the first Lifeboat Saturday. Next she took the initiative to organise the ladies of Manchester and Salford into committees with the purpose of raising further funds. Having secured the support of the Mayoresses of Manchester and of Salford, they were able to draw other influential women to volunteer help. Good networking skills were as valuable then as now.

Mrs Macara then responded to a letter that had been published in the Manchester press by Mr G. McConnel urging the women of England to support the lifeboats. She wrote:

> The earnest appeal to the women of England to help in the lifeboat cause which has been made by Mr E.G. McConnell [*sic*] of Manchester will, I feel sure, meet with an even more hearty response than his last year's one entitled 'Women and Children first'. The graphic way in which his own experience of seeing a life boat put out to sea in a whole gale against wind and tide must have touched many a woman's heart. I, too, have seen a lifeboat launched in a fearful storm, and have waited and watched with the wives and mothers of the crew, all through the long hours of a wild December night, for the return of the brave men who went out to save, but alas! returned no more.

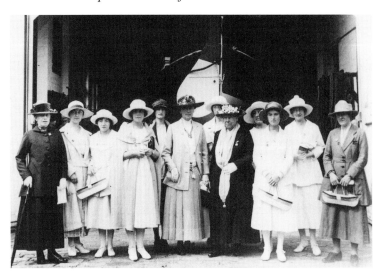

Lady Marion Macara (front row, right of centre) with the St Annes-on-Sea Ladies Lifeboat Guild, 1922. (Lytham Lifeboat Museum)

Such are the sacrifices which the humble homes of our fisher folk are called upon from time to time to make. Surely the wives and daughters of England will not be behind in doing their share towards the maintenance of this noble voluntary force. I am glad to see that Lady Roscoe is taking a lead in this matter. If a central committee of ladies could be organised in the North of England and another in the South, with subcommittees in each town to collect small sums from the many in aid of the Lifeboat Saturday Fund, I think it would be a great assistance in commencing the movement where it has not been taken up, and also in rendering permanent success.

Using an emotive argument and backing it up with great organisational skills, Marion Macara had effectively launched what was to become known as the Ladies' Lifeboat Auxiliary. In the November 1892 issue of the *Lifeboat Journal* it was announced:

It has been admirably suggested that Ladies' Committees should be formed in every county, city and town in Great Britain and Ireland for the purpose of raising funds for the Royal National Lifeboat Institution. All will agree that the idea is an excellent one, and we heartily commend it to all our lady supporters and friends, who will, we trust take immediate action in the matter. Do not wait to be asked to join such a committee, but take steps to organize one.

Thus was the mighty blessing of 'the men' given! It is unlikely that they knew what had been unleashed. The ladies were about to deploy their intelligence, skills and energies, much of which was inhibited by received wisdom and expectations of how women should fill their day, to raise funds for the lifeboat service. Many millions of pounds would accrue to the RNLI thanks to this collective power.

To achieve the objective of establishing so many Ladies' Auxiliary Committees, Marion Macara wrote many letters to well-connected ladies who might be persuaded to follow her lead. It was painstaking work, so how pleased she must have been to attract the interest of a journalist. Emily Faithfull had an article entitled 'WOMAN', published in *Lady's Pictorial* on 8 October 1892. It starts:

As some two thousand wrecks take place every year round our five thousand miles of coast, it must be allowed the appeal of the Lancashire ladies to their sisters throughout the British Isles is a timely one and Mrs Bosdin T. Leech, as Mayoress of Manchester, may be congratulated on having in that capacity initiated a movement which is destined to prove a national one. It may be confidently predicted that the ladies who occupy similar positions will be encouraged to join in the noble work of launching the best lifeboats which can be made for those who risk their lives to save their fellow creatures, and to provide for the widows and orphans that they leave behind them when such gallant efforts to save others from the perils of the sea end fatally, and the brave life-boat men share the fate of those they hoped to rescue from a watery grave.

Emily Faithfull goes on to acknowledge the work of Marion Macara to reach the consciences of more ladies, and then makes an observation which clearly reveals where on the social scale Mrs Macara was targeting her efforts:

> … her work was greatly increased by the fact that Lancashire is 'not at home' at this season of the year, but is to be found on Scottish moors and Swiss mountains, by the Cornish or Welsh coats – anywhere but in the neighbourhood of Cottonopolis.

She concludes her article with the strongest possible appeal to the hearts of her readers:

> … The wives, children and sweethearts of those brave fellows stood with white and tearful faces watching the scene, but to the glory of women it may be chronicled that not one word was uttered to deter husband, father or lover from setting forth on his perilous mission.
>
> As the women of England have little chance of being called upon to brave the fury of the winds and waves in efforts to save those who are battling for their lives on the open seas, they should at least do their utmost to secure an efficient service of life-boats.

An unequivocal call to action, which, together with all the others that issued from the Macara pen, brought outstanding results. Ladies' Auxiliary committees were formed

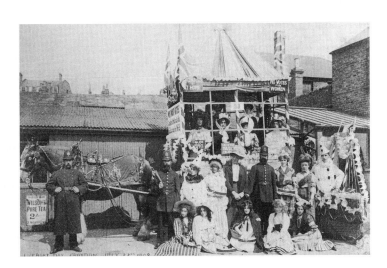

Postcard of Croydon Lifeboat Day, 1908. (Iain Booth postcard collection)

throughout the country, and as their fundraising activities grew, a stream of regular income made its way to the RNLI coffers. Ever a woman of action, Marion Macara undertook an onerous workload as the Honorary Secretary of Manchester Ladies' Council, which also coordinated the activities of thirty-one districts around the conurbation. In addition, she contributed in her hometown as President of St Anne's Committee.

Ladies' Lifeboat Auxiliary committees were established at many other lifeboat stations where there was an obvious affinity and loyalty between the women and the lifeboat crew. Numerically, though, the greatest number of committees was in inland locations, where passion for supporting the brave men who went out in open lifeboats risking their lives for others equalled that of those on the coast.

While Lifeboat Saturday remained an important and lucrative fundraising event for them, the ladies were quick to expand the repertoire. They were imaginative and resourceful, recognising the great chemistry of linking the pleasures of social events with securing money for a charitable cause – a formula that works very effectively today! Concerts, balls, luncheons, garden parties, fêtes and bazaars became the recognised way to have fun and fundraise. The good and the great were invited and were pleased to be seen supporting a good cause. Most committees had their local Mayoress installed as President, so there was usually a civic retinue in attendance too.

Marion Macara's strategy to secure leadership by the most influential ladies in the local community worked very effectively. In many places it was a sign of social acceptability and a privilege to be invited to join the committee, and ladies longed to receive their invitation. Seemingly some waited for years, but did not hesitate to accept when it finally came.

An interesting point is that, although the headquarters of the RNLI were in the capital, it took a little longer for the London ladies to form a committee. Not until August 1895 was a meeting called at Grosvenor House for the purpose of forming a ladies' committee in London. It was a successful rallying of the troops, though, as the *Lifeboat Journal* records in the November 1895 issue:

> …The fact that a strong and very influential committee of ladies has been formed with the express purpose of 'working the oracle' in London augurs well for life-boat interests in the metropolis.

Throughout the years of the First World War, the ladies continued as best they could to keep funds flowing in to sustain operation of the lifeboat service. The RNLI's finances were significantly affected by the war, and there was a real need to ensure that increased costs – the amount needed to run the service had reached £250,000 by 1921 – could be met by an increased income. It seems that the loyal ladies were to be the best solution.

Ladies' Lifeboat Guilds – developing a national network of fundraisers

With the underpinning idea of binding their loyalty even more tightly, it was announced in May 1921 that a Ladies' Lifeboat Guild was to be formed. This was launched by HRH the Prince of Wales at the annual meeting:

Thousands of women in every part of the United Kingdom, rich or poor, high or low, have shown that they are moved by the same spirit of mercy and helpfulness as actuated by Grace Darling. In their own way, they have rendered magnificent service to the Life-boat cause. Without them it would have been almost impossible to organise successfully those appeals, especially in the shape of life-boat day efforts, which bring the claims of the Institution to the sympathetic attention of the million. I feel sure that you and they will welcome the Institution's decision to form a bond of union among all these women in the establishment of the Ladies' Lifeboat Guild.

Essentially, the thinking was to give the ladies a greater sense of fellowship in their work. They were to have their own insignia in the form of a brooch, with a bar and a ribbon for office holders. A card of membership signed by the President would be presented to each lady. For this they had to 'have a readiness to help by *personal service* in the Guild's task of interesting and educating the public in the work of the Life-boat service, and of raising funds to maintain it'.

The Duchess of Portland, who already had a long record of support, had agreed to be President, and early on in her new role she sent a letter to all lifeboat stations urging their support for the Ladies' Lifeboat Guild:

> I think it will be an immense satisfaction and incentive to us all, in our work for this great cause, to feel we are united in a single body, and to know that, wherever we may go, we shall find new friends who are members of the Guild, and who have with us a common interest, duty and pleasure in its work.

The Guild was formally inaugurated at a meeting at Claridge's Hotel in June 1921, with all Presidents and Honourable Secretaries of Greater London Ladies' Auxiliary Committees invited. The Duchess expressed the hope that similar meetings would be held throughout the country.

Although the RNLI stated that it was not intended to alter in any way 'the excellent organisation of the Ladies' Auxiliaries', all office holders and members of the existing committees were automatically to become original members of the Guild. It may not have been their declared intention, but this initiative was to mark the demise of the Ladies' Auxiliary in favour of the Ladies' Lifeboat Guild.

Advice for the ladies was readily available. An article in the *Lifeboat Journal* in November 1921, written by an unnamed person who preferred to be known as 'a Life-boat Worker of Twenty-five Years' Experience', offered up their wisdom on 'one of the best and most inexpensive methods of making appeals – the "House to house" Collection'. She, or he, goes on to outline three possible ways of running a successful collection. The first involves delivering an envelope, 'showing the Wreck Chart of the British Isles with short concise facts about the Institution's work' to be collected the following day. The second method is by 'personal solicitation' and the merits are seen as being 'a happy way of interesting the "lady of the House" in the Institution's work and securing her as an Annual Subscriber'. Thirdly, a Collecting Card, which could be used by the householder to obtain personal contributions from their own friends and acquaintances. The article concludes by reassuring new Guild

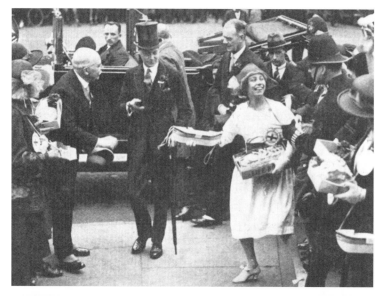

London Lifeboat Day, 1923. A hopeful collector greets the Prince of Wales at Lambeth Town Hall. (Central Press)

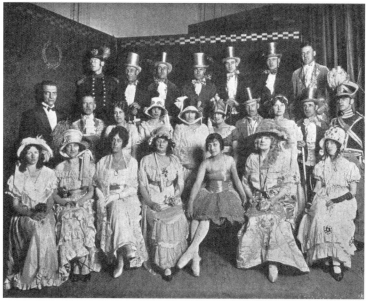

Eastbourne Centenary Ball, held in Devonshire Park, 1924. Everyone came dressed in 1824 costumes. (Frederick A. Bourne)

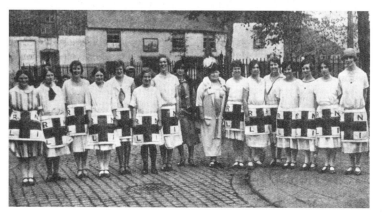

Carlisle, 1926. A fundraising event at the Café Chantant where all the volunteers wore an RNLI house flag apron. (*The Carlisle Journal*)

members that they will be 'received with sympathy and, in the great majority of cases, on obtaining an immediate response to their appeal'.

Civic support continued to be important in positioning the local Ladies' Lifeboat Guild at the heart of the community. Mayoresses almost always undertook the role of President, and it is clear that they took an active role in supporting organised events, seen to be very encouraging for the 'workers'. The importance of the royal and aristocratic patronage was very significant in these early days of the Ladies' Lifeboat Guild. In the interwar society, they brought status, influence, charisma, glamour and, of course, the promise of contributions from their own wealth.

In the role of President of the Guild, the Duchess of Portland was followed by HRH Princess Louise, Duchess of Argyll in 1924, and then by the Duchess of Sutherland in 1926. By this time the number of Guilds had expanded to:

North of England:	26
Midlands:	3
London District:	2
South-east England:	4
South-west England:	16
Scotland:	1
Ireland and Wales:	7
(Including Hereford and Shropshire)	

The centenary of the RNLI in 1924 was celebrated everywhere. Encouraged to rejoice in 100 years of saving lives at sea – and raise more funds – the volunteers responded with a prodigious range of special events, both at the coast and far inland. They included concerts, garden parties, lifeboat demonstrations, dinners, carnivals, and balls. Many communities organised services of thanksgiving; in Manchester this had to be held in the Royal Exchange, as it was the only building in the city that would hold so large a congregation. In the Midlands there was a motor tour pulling a modern lifeboat, which passed through sixteen counties, taking nearly six months to complete. A Centenary Supplement was produced in the *Lifeboat Journal* and special souvenirs were produced which were available for the ladies' guilds to sell.

During the presidency of the Duchess of Sutherland it was agreed to inaugurate a General Council, which would coordinate the activities of the increasing number of Guilds. The first meeting was held at her home in Green Street, London, and was attended by HRH the Prince of Wales. The Duchess opened the proceedings with a feisty speech, urging the ladies to overcome the 'enemy' of 'apathy and ignorance' among the general public towards the lifeboat cause. She then invited her VIP guest to speak:

> ... At the last Annual Meeting, the Institution honoured the women of Boulmer, in Northumberland, as it has honoured the women of Holy Island and many another little fishing village for their devoted services in assisting to launch the life-boat under circumstances of the greatest difficulty and danger, many a time going into the water waist high in their anxiety to ensure a prompt and successful launch ... the work of thousands of women in organising the

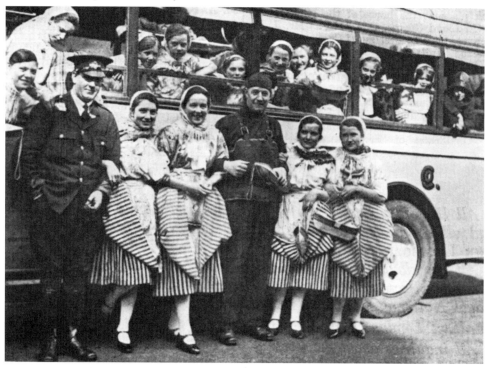

Fisher girls in the procession at Edinburgh Lifeboat Day, 1932. (*The Glasgow Bulletin*)

thankless task of raising funds for this great Institution has been carried on in the same spirit and with magnificent results. I am told that fully two thirds of the amount raised annually for the Institution in connection with Life-boat day efforts, fêtes, bazaars, house to house collections etc is due to the work of women, and I should like to pay a warm tribute to the large numbers of those who have recognised in the Life-boat Service a Cause which represents not only the courage and endurance of our race, but especially its humanity and kindness of heart … the times are not easy for those who take up charitable and philanthropic work, and work for the life-boat Cause is, perhaps, more than usually arduous because great and overwhelming as are its claims, it requires a strong effort of the imagination on the part of the ordinary man in the street to realise the services that are carried out on some remote spot on the coast in the darkness on a winter's night … I place the Lifeboat Cause in your hands, confident that it is safe with you as the life-boat is safe in the hands of our gallant crews.

This extract from his speech, published in the *Lifeboat Journal* in February 1927, concludes with the note that it was greeted with loud cheers. The Prince had filled the ladies with renewed enthusiasm and motivation to do yet more. The result was several more years of continuing growth in the number of committees, an ever-expanding repertoire of fund-raising activities, and a healthy flow of income.

Patricia Kellehar at seventeen years old.

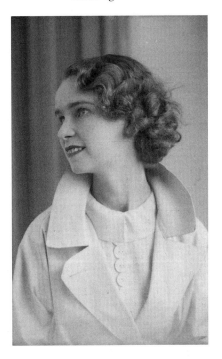

Children on board

Understanding that, if encouraged young, children are more likely to become adult lifeboat supporters, the Duke of Northumberland initiated a national lifeboat essay competition which ran each year from 1918 to 1939. The subject was the same every time.

Patricia Kellehar from Sussex, now aged ninety-one, won the competition in 1932. She was aged thirteen when she wrote this essay.

<u>Qualities which make a good life-boat man</u>
We read in history books of the famous men and women who gave their lives for their fellow men, but do we ever think of the life-boat men, of how they rescue hundreds and hundreds of lives? Many a lifeboat man feels proud when he tells the stories of how he rescued many and many a person, when the ship was almost swallowed up by the green ocean.

The lifeboat-man needs a great deal of courage, for instance, supposing on a dark and stormy night about two o'clock the life-boatman was called out to go to mid-ocean and rescue the people on a sinking ship, it would not be very pleasant would it. But he thinks not of himself but of his fellow men, of how he will rescue those who if it were not for him would be swallowed up by the raging seas. A life-boatman too has to have spirit to overcome his difficulties and to do his work with a good heart.

We must not forget that when those gallant men set out to sea they are risking their own lives and what are their wives and children going to do if they are killed. The Royal National Lifeboat Institution sees to that; they provide for the wife and children.

To qualify as a life-boatman a man must be healthy, strong and sturdy and able to fight against any rough weather. A life-boatman should be a man who can keep his head like this passage from Rudyard Kipling 'If you can keep your head when all about you are losing theirs and blaming it on you, you'll be a man my son'.

A man too, if he wants to be a life-boatman should be alert and quick in action.

There are many qualities has but the main point is he should be courageous. If a man cannot swim he is not much use as a life-boatman, as often the boat will overturn and all the men will be tipped out. A life-boatman is a brave man and deserves a great deal of praise.

The Duke of Northumberland's idea worked – Patricia supported the RNLI throughout her life and encouraged her son, Paul, to do the same. A keen deep-sea yachtsman, he is a volunteer RNLI Safety Adviser delivering the SEA Check service to boaters.

Post-war challenges – recruiting and retaining volunteers

Throughout the Second World War, the fundraisers worked on. Many fewer fundraising events were held, but most of the committees organised lifeboat days. These returned a lower income than formerly, but were still an important source of money to keep the service running.

Post-war years brought huge societal changes, and with more women in employment, the supply of willing housewives to join committees dwindled. The RNLI realised that it would have to work even harder to secure women volunteers. Much more than the influence of the good and the great was now needed, and a new personal touch was provided through a network of paid staff whose task it was to recruit and retain volunteers for both ladies' guilds and financial branches.

Isabella Morison, District Organising Secretary and Regional Coordinator

Isabella Morison had the same insight as Marion Macara – when seeking help it is best to go straight to the top. When she started employment with the RNLI in 1950, she had a big challenge to increase the number of fundraising committees and so increase voluntary income for the RNLI from north-east England. Wherever a new committee was needed, she went to the influential people in that area and, with their contacts, drew together people who would help. Realising that women were already doing the majority of fundraising, she concentrated her energies on recruiting the help of men.

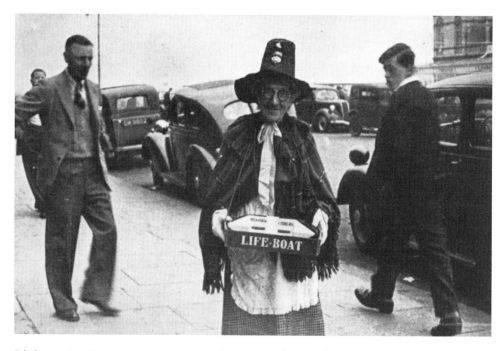

Rhyl, 1949. Mrs Davenport, aged ninety-one, has collected in her traditional Welsh costume for twenty-one years.

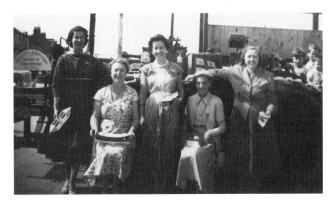

Isabella Morrison (on the far left)
collecting at Redcar in 1959.

When in inland communities, her technique was to 'take the sea to them' by speaking in a direct and knowledgeable way about the realities of the lifeboat service. To do this effectively she needed to get to know the lifeboat stations and the crews very well. She regularly visited them all and took the opportunity of the routine training exercises to join the crew on the lifeboat so that she could gain a first-hand understanding of all that they did to save lives at sea. Then when she was appealing for help in places such as Bradford or Leeds, she could bring it all alive for her audience.

Working with volunteers brings many challenges and, now aged ninety-five, Isabella recalls how important it was to have the skills of tact and diplomacy. There were times when she was called upon to keep the peace. The important thing was to concentrate on the needs of the RNLI, especially when the income was not keeping pace with expenditure. It was this situation that brought her a promotion to the position of North Region Coordinator. Her task was to provide direction and support amongst the RNLI branches and guilds for the initiatives being generated at Headquarters to increase the income flow. For the RNLI, her experience was invaluable, and for Isabella it was just the kind of challenge she relished. Having almost failed to get the job when she first applied in 1950, she retired in 1976 with the feeling that she and the RNLI 'were meant to be'.

A loyal female colleague Isabella remembers well was Mary Lloyd Jones, who was the District Organising Secretary for Scotland from 1958 until 1981. Mary immediately joined Isabella in County Durham to go and give support to the families of the five crew members of Seaham lifeboat who were tragically drowned while on service in November 1962. Mary was to have this sad duty again in Scotland, when in 1967 at Longhope eight crew members were drowned, and in 1970 at Fraserburgh when a further five succumbed to the same cruel fate.

Christine Oliver – catching your volunteers young!

One person who can testify to the persuasive powers of a RNLI District Organising Secretary seeking to raise money for the RNLI is Christine Oliver. When she was just sixteen years old and then Christine Ford living in Portslade, she was visited by Mrs Robinson who, explaining that there was no local RNLI Branch, 'asked' if she would like to form one. And so it was that Christine, having only just left school, became the youngest ever Ladies' Lifeboat Guild Honorary Secretary.

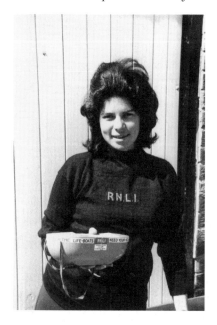

Christine Oliver collecting in Salisbury with a brand new plastic collecting box, *c.*1970.

Her interest in lifeboats had begun, aged thirteen, on a family holiday in Devon. Her father took great delight in hunting out lifeboat stations in the West Country and Christine enjoyed the fact that many of them were situated in interesting coves or towns. When Christine was encouraged by a crew member at Selsey to write to RNLI HQ, she did not hesitate, and it was that letter which brought Mrs Robinson to her front door. So in 1957, Portslade Ladies' Lifeboat Guild was formed with the help of friends and relations, including best friend Rosemary and six-year-old cousin Rene. The earliest fundraising activity was a 'Salvage Drive'. Leaflets were delivered requesting clothes, bric-a-brac and even jam jars, which could then be sold for a farthing. The Guild went from strength to strength with bazaars, house-to-house collections, Flag Days, carol singing, and collections of silver paper and milk bottle tops.

It was at an RNLI event that Christine met her husband to be – a young man named Anthony Oliver who belonged to RNLI Hurstpierpoint Branch. They married in 1964, and theirs was the first wedding picture to feature in the *Lifeboat Journal*. Married life was closely interwoven with fundraising, as they became joint Honorary Secretaries of Basingstoke and District Branch. A baby girl arrived just over a year later and her lifeboat-coloured navy blue pram was covered in flags for Flag Day. In 1966 Anthony joined the RNLI staff, meaning that they had to move to Weston-super-Mare. Here Christine became Lifeboat Week organiser – ensuring that every road in the town was covered was a huge task, but a very lucrative one.

A later move to Salisbury brought more opportunities to fundraise. By now they had two small children and both were involved. Christine has vivid memories of combining her role as a mother with RNLI activities:

> As a family we went with Anthony to Boat Shows, Agricultural Shows and the Steam Fair, armed with a huge picnic basket which the children raided continuously. Loads of extra clothes – they always fell in the water or mud, whichever was available. We always lost the children while I helped sell Lottery tickets or souvenirs alongside Anthony. They scrounged food from the cookery demonstrations, tormented the army and their guns, collected the deposit money on the beer glasses that they sneaked away from unsuspecting drinkers and were occasionally brought back looking absolutely filthy, only to run off again.

Her last official RNLI volunteer role was as Flag Week organiser for Broadstone Branch. She retired on moving to Wimborne in 1984. By this time she had given twenty-seven years' continuous service. This was recognised in the same year when she was presented

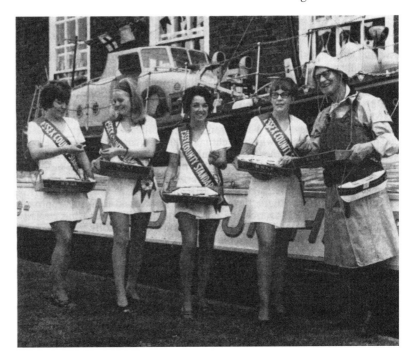

Colchester Flag Day, 1970. *Essex County Standard* employees lend a hand. (*Essex County Standard*)

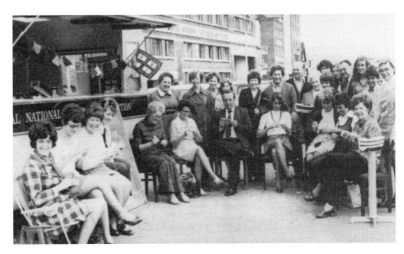

Poole, 1974. To support the fundraisers, RNLI employees held lunch-hour sponsored knit-ins. (*Times Herald* Newspapers)

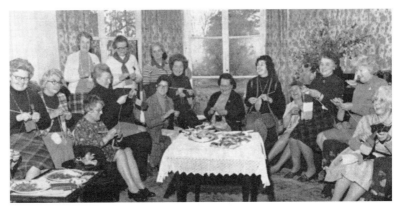

Tamworth Ladies Guild, 1976. A knit-in held in the home of the Guild Chairman. (J. Walker)

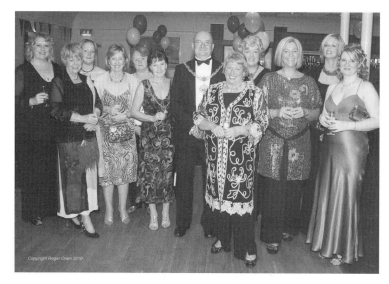

Douglas Ladies Guild at their dinner dance in 2007. (Roger Oram)

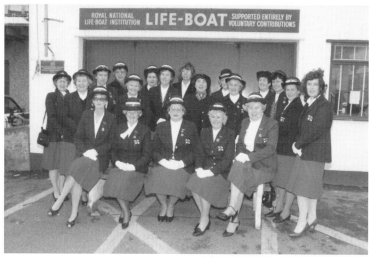

Newquay Ladies Guild – instantly recognisable in their uniform.

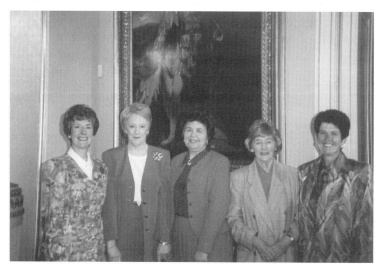

Liverpool Ladies Guilds – members of the organising committee for the 'Successful Women of Merseyside' luncheons, 1995.

with a Gold Badge by HRH the Duchess of Kent at the Festival Hall. For both Christine and Anthony, there was a special pride in the fact that this was one of the first awards given to the wife of a staff member.

Further post-war challenges – reserves are nearly depleted

Operationally and financially, the post-war years presented huge challenges for the RNLI with the volunteer fundraisers once again providing a crucial source of support to achieve the ambitious aim to expand and modernise the fleet. With the reserves at worryingly low levels for several years in the early 1970s, encouragement was given to the ladies' guilds and financial branches to increase their efforts. This was met with an enthusiastic response – for many volunteers the prospect of having to seek Government help was quite unthinkable. Committees throughout the United Kingdom and Republic of Ireland were urged to be even more active. The outcome was a flow of raised voluntary income, which continued to rise year on year.

Just as the RNLI had pushed the boat out to celebrate its 100th anniversary, many of the ladies' guilds and financial branches used their formation dates as special silver and golden anniversaries – to raise additional funds and to have some fun by hosting a party. By the 1990s, centenaries started to be celebrated. Marion Macara's own committee, St Anne's Ladies' Lifeboat Guild, was the first guild to reach this milestone in 1993. They organised a summer ball, and received commemorative vellum.

Doing it their way

Ladies lifeboat guilds and financial branches everywhere share an identical purpose – raising funds to support the lifeboat crews. The passion and pride of volunteer fundraisers in supporting these courageous volunteer lifesavers has been a consistent element in the chemistry of the organisation for over a century. All over the country – in places far inland as well as on the coast – the talents and skills of many thousands of women have resulted in many millions of pounds raised to fund the lifeboat service. The word 'tireless' to describe volunteers may well have become overworked, but within the RNLI committee network it is still possible to meet hundreds of women who are just that – tireless in their commitment, loyalty and enterprise to support the cause. It would be a vast undertaking to document them all – but attend any fundraising event and you will see RNLI women in action and readily recognise their qualities.

All committees use the RNLI-branded fundraising materials to ensure that public presentation of the organisation is accurate and consistent. This is well understood as good practice, but up and down the country individuality in style and tradition has developed among the groups, which means that no two are the same. There being 1,347 committees in total, it would be impossible to describe them all, and so here is just a flavour of their diversity.

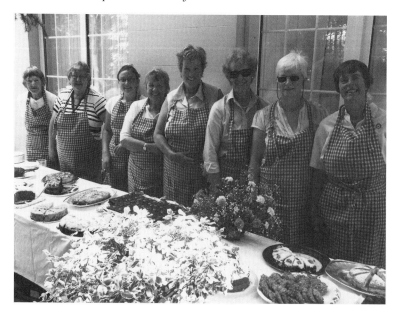

Jersey Ladies' Guild – renowned for their excellent cooking.

On the Isle of Man, the home of Sir William Hillary, and where commitment to the RNLI runs deep, there are five Ladies' Guilds linked with each lifeboat station: Douglas, Peel, Ramsey, Port St Mary and Port Erin. Lifeboat station committees on the island have always been particularly active in fundraising, but they drew upon the support of women long before the Ladies' Guilds were formed, which appears to be somewhat later here than elsewhere.

Lifeboat Days and Flag Days have long been major sources of income. In the days when the Isle of Man was a popular holiday destination, collectors positioned themselves at the ferry terminal to good effect. During the traditional 'wakes weeks' when thousands of people came from Scotland and Lancashire, the best places to collect were in the pubs. In the 1950s, some women would go up into the hills to pick heather to make into posies to sell, while others picked roses from their gardens to make into button holes – both secured a much larger donation than a paper flag! In Port St Mary, cornflowers were grown to sell on Lifeboat Day.

With each guild organising a programme of events, the residents of the Isle of Man are presented with many opportunities to support their lifeboat service, which they do with great generosity. For many years the amount of money raised per head of population has exceeded anywhere else within the RNLI. In 2009 alone, this was almost £167,000.

Newquay Ladies' Lifeboat Guild in Cornwall is very distinctive. They have developed their own 'uniform' making them instantly recognisable when they take advantage of a wide range of local events such as carnivals and air days to fundraise. In north Cornwall their cream teas have a very special reputation. Chairman, Pauline Morris, cannot be sure how many they have made over the years – many hundreds, no doubt!

In Liverpool, where there were a number of ladies' guilds, someone had the idea of forming the Liverpool and District Ladies' Guilds. With its own Chairman it would ensure coordination and support of all the other committees. Throughout the 1960s, '70s and '80s this worked well, with each committee specialising in the events that worked best in their part of Merseyside. Each year the ladies met for an AGM, held variously on one of the ships in Liverpool Docks, on HMS *Eaglet*, and then at venues around the district.

The real strength of this federation was demonstrated when a decision was made in 1995 to organise a series of luncheons in Liverpool Town Hall with the theme 'Successful Women of Merseyside'. All the organisational and ticket-selling skills of the separate guilds was called upon to achieve success.

The speakers were all from Merseyside or had achieved their success there: Rosie Cooper, youngest Lord Mayor of Liverpool; Elaine Griffiths, the first female cardiothoracic surgeon; Baroness Linda Chalker, politician; Judge Elizabeth Steele; and Patricia Routledge, actress. So successful was the series that a second was held the following year, with Judith Greensmith, Chair of Merseyside Health Authority, Penny Hughes, former President of Coca Cola, and Pauline Daniels, actress. The whole series raised £20,000.

By 2006 the number of guilds had greatly declined, so it was decided to bring the Liverpool and District Ladies' Guilds to a close. In her final speech, Ann Walker, who had been Chairman for fifteen years, confirmed that they had raised the wonderful sum of £908,775 during that period.

As far south as the RNLI map goes is Jersey Ladies' Lifeboat Guild, which, in 1932, the first year it was founded, raised £100. In 2009, the ladies raised £100,000! There are sixty-three members of the Guild, some of whom help regularly and others when they can. Their fundraising programme comprises the traditional mix of events that people love to attend and they have a shop in St Helier Lifeboat Station that opens thanks to a rota of helpers from Easter to Christmas. A shrewd move has been to involve other organisations on the island to fundraise for the RNLI – the Band of the Island of Jersey, St Quen Artists group and the Total Sport Half Marathon have all helped. Renowned as good cooks, much of their most successful fundraising also involves food, for which their customers come back time and time again.

It is hardly surprising that their proximity to the lifeboat station and crew is very motivating for the guild members, and they speak proudly of the particular pleasure it has given them to fundraise for the pagers that summon their crew for launching the lifeboat. Similarly, they worked really hard to help contribute to the £1.3 million appeal for a new Tamar class lifeboat for the station.

Now known as Central London Committee, it was first formed in 1917 as the London Ladies' Committee and was given the responsibility for organising Flag Day collections. The first committee included: Mrs Lloyd George, wife of the Prime Minister; Lady Waldegrave, wife of the Chairman of the RNLI Committee of Management; and the wives of Admirals Jellicoe and Beatty. It was able to use the Headquarters of the RNLI for meetings. A new constitution was adopted in 1923 in which the name was stated to be The London Women's Committee.

At first the main fundraising activity centred upon London Lifeboat Day, and the task of the committee was to organise collecting depots throughout the capital and to ensure that there were as many collectors as possible on the streets. It was conducted with an almost military precision and was extremely lucrative. However, the success of a variety matinee

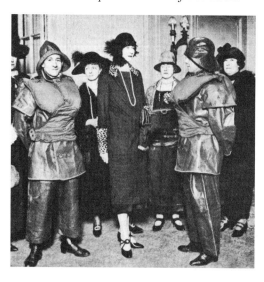

The Duchess of Sutherland opening the London Bazaar at the Hyde Park Hotel. Held on 3 and 4 March 1925, it marked the end of the centenary year and the RNLI's 101st birthday. (Keystone View Co.)

performance at the Hippodrome, attended by King George IV and Queen Mary, encouraged members to expand their repertoire of fundraising activities into social events. This was to become their speciality.

Throughout the war years the committee met regularly. Amazingly, the minutes of these meetings make scant reference to the hostilities – the focus remained strong and true to supporting the RNLI. One of the references made in 1941 was when, after discussion, it was agreed that their customary 'winter effort' would have to be postponed because of the difficulty in selling tickets when so many members were out of London. A garden party at St James, with the Duchess of Kent as guest of honour, was planned for 1945. Sadly, that too had to be postponed. Lifeboat Days did continue throughout the war, though – the one in 1942 raised £20,477 16s. 11d.

In the past sixty years, the committee has grown and now has forty-five members, many of whom are active and adventurous sailors. Most have long experience of fundraising. Their immensely practical and original ideas are aired robustly at monthly meetings to guide the nine annual events they present, each run by an event committee headed by its own Chairman. Their direct contribution from these events to the RNLI is generally between £250,000 and £300,000 per annum.

The principal event in the Central London calendar is a ball or banquet which takes place in the winter, and aims to raise a six-figure sum. To their delight, in the cash-strapped year of 2009 their Yellow Welly Party at Hurlingham Club raised a record of over £158,000. Other regular events include a Golf Day, a Men's Tennis Tournament at Queen's Club, a private view of marine art at the Mall Galleries, a Winter Luncheon in the Royal Thames Yacht Club and a Bridge Afternoon in Pont Street Church Hall, where homemade teas are prepared for almost 200 players.

Why do these events make thousands where many similar charities make hundreds? The committee would say it is the constancy and generosity of their close friends and supporters, who attend, sponsor, act as guest speakers, give valuable prizes, and don't hesitate to bid for them too. The inexorable rise of the Auction Prize, whose electronic bidding system

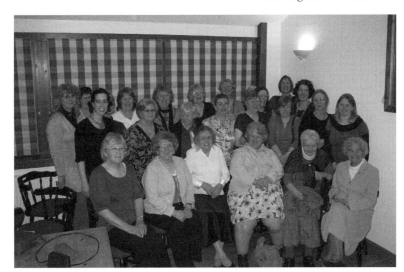

Longhope Ladies Guild celebrating their 50th anniversary in 2010.

provides night-long excitement without interrupting the general enjoyment, is making a huge impact on fundraising everywhere. Flag Day also continues to be a cornerstone of their fundraising, giving the man in the street few chances to ignore the collecting boxes flourished from dawn to dusk at railway stations, clubs, arts venues and street corners.

The fundraising year concludes with a carol service, with lessons often read by guests from The Royal Navy, The Port of London Authority, Trinity House and lifeboat crew. This is free to all and gives the committee an opportunity to celebrate Christmas and enjoy a drink with their many friends and supporters.

Possibly the most remote community in which there is a Ladies' Guild is Longhope on Hoy in the Orkney Islands. The island has a population of less than 400 people and twenty-three of these are members of the guild. The ladies explain that the lifeboat station, crew and guild are part of the fabric of island life and they receive outstanding support from the community, which well understands the need for a lifeboat service. Throughout the summer season the lifeboat shop is an important source of income, but the ladies will willingly open it at any other time of the year if requested. Popular events include the Christmas bazaar, bingo and skittles nights, and on Lifeboat Day, the cream teas are a speciality. A favourite recipes book sells well too.

The lifeboat station is the perfect place for their regular meetings and the crew are always willing to help with the heavy lifting jobs at fundraising events. It is this willingness to support each other that lies at the heart of the lifeboat people at Longhope, who know all too well the terrible price that may sometimes be paid when a lifeboat launches to the rescue of others. The entire crew of eight men were lost when the Longhope lifeboat capsized on service in March 1969 and were caught by the raging sea. Their wives have grieved privately and with great dignity, but resolutely continued in their support for the Longhope lifeboat cause.

Cullercoats Fishwives

They were never an official RNLI fundraising group but their work to raise money for the service has been legendary. It all started in 1922 when twenty-six of the local fishwives in Cullercoats, dressed in their traditional costume of layered skirts and richly coloured silk shawls, each took a collecting box around the community on the occasion of the quarterly summer exercise of Cullercoats lifeboat. They collected £60 and decided to do the same thing the following year – and so began a tradition which was to last for almost fifty years.

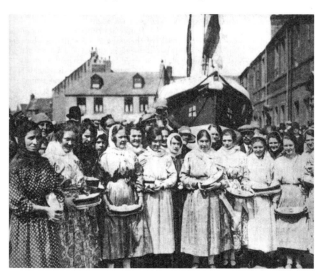

The fishwives of Cullercoats, 1923.

Soon the number of fish-wives willing to take part rose to sixty, and to add to the sense of occasion, they organised for a local band to come and play, paying for their services from their own pockets and providing them with tea. Each year the sum collected rose.

In the early days the most successful collector was Polly Donkin. She was awarded the RNLI Gold Brooch by The Prince of Wales in 1930. When he asked her the secret of her success, she replied: 'I *like* to get the money and I *get* the money' – a woman of few words, but much determination! Collections continued throughout the war years and by the end of 1945, the women had collected £4,620 since starting twenty-three years earlier.

The most successful collector of all time was Bella Mattison, and when she died in 1971 she was the last Cullercoats fishwife. By then she had personally collected over £8,000, earning her the description of 'a branch of the RNLI herself'. She became well known as 'Bella – the Lifeboat Lady'; people wanted to meet her and photograph her in the traditional costume. She travelled widely to events to display her shawls and, of course, to collect a fee that she then donated to the RNLI. She was awarded an RNLI Gold Brooch and was extremely proud to be a special guest to meet the Queen and Prince Philip when they visited the north-east coast.

Bella Mattison in 1951. (Northern Press Ltd)

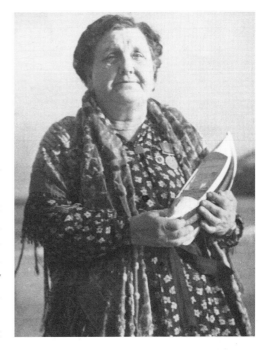

Thanks and recognition

Thanking its volunteers and giving recognition for service is something that the
RNLI knows to be vitally important. The
annual Presentation of Awards ceremony
is the occasion when the awards for gallantry are traditionally made to lifeboat
crew members – and what better occasion
to recognise the contribution made by the
fundraisers? It is a moving sight to see so
many women who have given fifty years'
– and more – service walk across the stage
to receive their award. Sometimes this
may be with some physical difficulty, but
never without pride and dignity. Citations
speak not only of what each has done to raise funds, but also of their personal qualities as
inspirational leaders, motivators and great organisers, demonstrating total reliability and
commitment.

Records of honorary awards have been kept since 1928 and since then, 10,627 women
have received them – more than half of all awards made by the RNLI in that period.

Raising funds in the twenty-first century

Many women fundraisers speak of what a pleasure it is to raise money for the RNLI. The
public is usually very supportive of a charity that has volunteers on the front line, risking
their lives to save others. Collecting house-to-house or on a Flag Day usually brings some
heart-warming stories of people who have been rescued, or why the RNLI is admired.
To hear this helps greatly when feet and legs are beginning to hurt after hours of standing
in the street or in the shopping mall. Some women become known locally as the 'lifeboat
lady' and there are apocryphal stories of how, seeing a woman valiantly collecting in the
rain, a person has been motivated to make a large donation or leave a legacy to the RNLI,
such was the respect for their commitment.

The number of Ladies' Lifeboat Guilds has declined significantly in recent years. The lack
of availability of younger women to undertake fundraising within a committee structure
has meant that some guilds have closed down, as their ageing membership felt unable to
continue. Some guilds, recognising their inability to recruit younger women, made the
decision to include men in the membership and become a financial branch. Happily, some
have succeeded in maintaining their numbers and continue to raise considerable sums of
money each year.

Running for the RNLI – the Bath Half-Marathon.

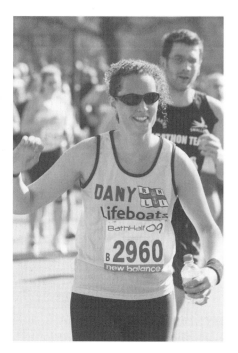

The RNLI is not alone in having declining numbers of fundraising committees – other charities are experiencing the same trend. Replacing this regular and reliable income stream is a major challenge, which the RNLI has met in a range of different ways, including sponsored events, the introduction of a national fundraising day, and youth fundraising.

Lifeboat courage of a different sort

Ask any RNLI fundraiser why they do it and they will speak of their respect and admiration for the brave lifeboat crews. Fundraisers are not without courage themselves, though, as was shown in 1996.

It was 15 June, the date of the Manchester Flag Day. It was also the day when the IRA bombed the city centre. I was myself running the collecting depot in Manchester Town Hall that day and there were around twenty people with collecting boxes on the streets, but the story is best told by one of the collectors, Betty Lockhart, from RNLI Stockport Branch, who was caught in the blast:

> Saturday was a lovely day and I decided to stand outside the Kendal Milne store – a good collection spot. I positioned myself at the corner nearest to Marks and Spencers. Suddenly there were policemen instructing people to move. I could also hear, from people talking all around me, that there could be a bomb in Manchester. There was no panic but obviously great apprehension. A policeman suggested that as I had a captive audience I should take advantage of it and go round with my collecting box!
>
> Simultaneously, with the bomb going off, the windows in the big building opposite Kendals seemed to bow and then they fell out. Suddenly Kendal's windows exploded and there was screaming and shouting. Glass was everywhere. I saw quite a number of people injured with flying and falling glass. Where I had been first standing I saw a lady with quite bad injuries. I saw two young girls, neither was injured but one was quite upset so I went and talked quietly to them. Then very quickly a helicopter appeared, flying very low and over a loud speaker there were shouts to the crowd to 'Run! Run!' indicating away from the city centre.
>
> The injured were being helped but many like me followed the helicopter instructions. I can remember feeling not panicked but very stressed and I knew I had to get to the Town Hall. I have never run so fast! I worried about the other collectors and if they were safe …

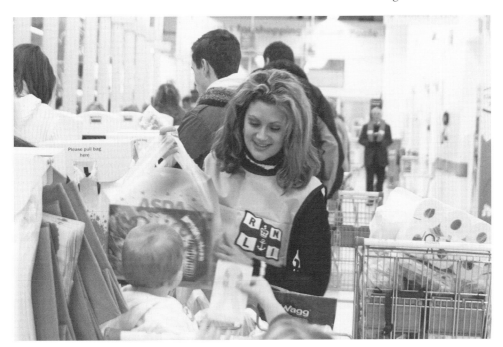

Packing bags at ASDA – RNLI staff help fundraise on SOS Day, 2008.

When Betty arrived back she was covered in glass – in her hair and over her face and clothes. She was shining with glass, but she was safe. As were all the other RNLI collectors, and how very brave they were, making no fuss and helping to get the money to a safe place before making for home. It was a day when their stoicism certainly matched what they so admire in the crews.

Many years previously in 1921, some ladies collecting in Dublin were caught in another dangerous situation. There was fighting on the streets and several members of the public were wounded. Some of the RNLI ladies had narrow escapes, and one rendered first aid to a woman who had fainted. The report in *the Lifeboat* goes on to say: 'The same lady helpers are nevertheless continuing to sell flags, and we are doing very well in the special effort generally.' Such are the extraordinary qualities of the women of the RNLI!

The qualities of commitment, loyalty, hard work and yes, courage, in the women fund-raisers are recognised and valued throughout the lifeboat service. It was a coxswain, though, who summarised their contribution perfectly. In his memorable address at the 1974 annual Presentation of Awards ceremony, Coxswain Derek Scott of the Mumbles lifeboat said:

> From the time the lady sold her flag or arranged her coffee morning to raise funds – that is when the rescue started and not when the maroons were fired. Anybody who works for or supports this Institution in some way is responsible for the preservation of life at sea.

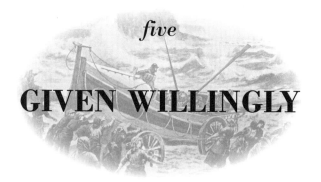

five

GIVEN WILLINGLY

Not everyone chooses to join a committee as a means of supporting the RNLI, preferring to 'do their own thing'. Women have found many different ways to do this: by leaving a legacy, making donations in their lifetime, fundraising individually, helping to save the RNLI's heritage, or through promotion of the RNLI's work.

The sum of individual generosity from women is so huge that it is impossible to capture completely within one publication. This sample conveys an idea of how much, whether of time or of money, women have given willingly.

I bequeath …

On a wall in RNLI Headquarters is a wooden plaque that always pulls my heartstrings whenever I walk past it. It reads:

The Trustees of the Will
of the late
Mrs Elizabeth Kirkham
Of Southport
gave the sum of £368.8.8 from her
estate to the funds of
The Royal National Lifeboat Institution
In memory of
Mrs Elizabeth Kirkham
And her four deceased children
1926

Mrs Kirkham is just one of many thousands of people who have written the RNLI into their will. Their motives for doing so are many and various, and not always known. What is certain is that legacies form a very important element of the annual income needed to run the lifeboat service. It is calculated that six out of every ten lifeboat launches are made possible because of legacy gifts.

Doris M. Mann

Doris Mann lived in Ampthill, Bedfordshire, which is a long way from the sea, and so it is perhaps surprising that she should leave a legacy to provide a lifeboat. The only child of a prominent builder, she committed her whole life to charitable causes and community service. The list of her involvement is lengthy, and includes: the Women's Institute; the Red Cross; Ampthill Servicemen's Club; Feoffee Almshouses; and the Church. She served on both the local district council and the county council for many years.

At some point the RNLI caught her interest and she involved herself with the local fundraising branch. It was her father's business interests that took her to Wells-next-the-Sea, where he owned a number of properties. One of their tenants was a fisherman and also a member of the local lifeboat crew. He took Doris out in a dinghy, giving her great pleasure but also, no doubt, information about their work at the lifeboat station. The other friendships she made among the lifeboat community meant much to her.

Her legacy provided for the lifeboat that entered service at Wells-next-the-Sea in 1990 – *Doris M. Mann of Ampthill.*

Mrs Ann Ritchie

When Ann Gough went to the Isle of Man to take up the post of Physical Training Supervisor for Schools, she planned to stay for just four years. Meeting James Ball Ritchie changed those plans, and after they had married she lived on the island for the rest of her life. The young couple shared a love of the sea and, thanks to the growing prosperity of Jim's family business, Heron and Brearley, in 1960 they commissioned the building of a motor yacht named *Silver Lal*, which gave them much pleasure as they cruised through the Clyde and Western Isles each summer.

By the late '60s the Ritchies were planning a new boat for themselves, and it was then that Jim learned of the proposed new lifeboat for Ramsey Lifeboat Station. He told his wife that he wanted to provide the funds for it, as he had long wanted to do something significant to help the RNLI. The donation was made, but sadly he died before the Oakley class lifeboat entered service in 1970. Ann proudly named it *James Ball Ritchie* in his memory. She avidly read the reports of the services by Ramsey and decided to provide funds for the new Arun class lifeboat scheduled to enter service at Port St Mary in 1977. The name she chose, *Gough Ritchie*, made the link between her own family and Jim's.

Ann had made the brave decision to take delivery of *Silver Lal* and to go to sea again with a hired crew. She did this for several years, cruising to Norway, France and Scotland. In 1983, she gave the money for a new lifeboat for Oban and named her *Alice Ann Ritchie*. This particular lifeboat had a short life because of problems that developed in the material used to build the hull. Ann was extremely distressed to learn this, but her response was a typically generous one – she made a substantial donation to the fund held by the RNLI for the benefit of widows and orphans of lifeboat crew. The Ladies' Lifeboat Guild at Ramsey was happy to welcome Ann as their President and she was keen to have a personal involvement in their fundraising activities. She spent her last fourteen years living in Ramsey and enjoyed the close friendship with the lifeboat community there and at other stations on the island.

Ann died in 1990 and, under the terms of her will, the residue of her estate became the Gough Ritchie Charitable Trust. One third of its annual income is distributed to the

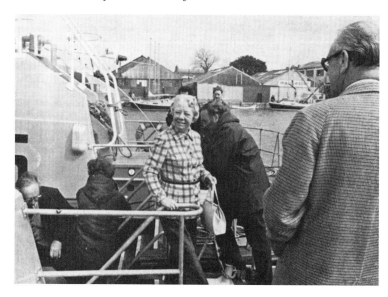

Ann Ritchie
on a visit to
Osbornes Boatyard,
Littlehampton, in
1976 to view the
Arun class lifeboat,
to be named *Gough
Ritchie*, which she
funded for Port
St Mary Lifeboat
Station.

RNLI for use on the Isle of Man. In the past twenty years it has helped to meet the costs of two more lifeboats – the *Ann and James Ritchie* at Ramsey, and the *Gough Ritchie II* at Port St Mary.

A generous lady who said she considered herself very lucky because she had been able to do what she really wanted to do – make a positive contribution to saving lives at sea. She claimed that her reward and her pleasure were in the pride of the crew in the Ritchie lifeboats, and the care they give them.

Margaret Ellen Foster

Margaret was born in Emsworth, Hampshire, and lived in the family home that faced the sea. Her father had a shipbuilding business and also traded in coal and timber. She was one of four children, none of whom married. They lived a quiet life Emsworth, but took a real interest in all matters relating to ships and the sea. So it was that Margaret chose to support the fundraising work of the local RNLI fundraising branch.

Margaret was the last surviving member of her family, and she died in 1995. Her will made provision for a number of charities, including the RNLI. Her legacy was used to provide a new lifeboat for Kirkwell in the Orkneys, a place far from Emsworth, but her executors felt that she would be very happy to provide a lifeboat for a place where the sea is so dangerous. The lifeboat *Margaret Foster* went to Kirkwall in 2008, where she carries out long and arduous services.

Susan Hiscock MBE

It is not clear when Susan made her decision to leave a substantial legacy to the RNLI, but when she died in 1995 her will revealed that, after specific bequests, the residue of her estate was to go to the RNLI to provide a lifeboat to be named *Wanderer*. This was the name she and her husband, Eric, had given to all five yachts they had jointly owned between 1941 and 1986.

Susan Hiscock on board *Wanderer II* in the late 1940s.

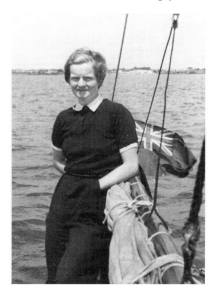

Susan and Eric had developed a highly distinctive lifestyle on their yachts, sailing around the world a total of three times – not in an endeavour to break speed records, but to experience different places and people in slow time. Each voyage took up to three years, during which they made many friends who found the couple's independent minded-ness and sailing skills quite inspirational. They were the first husband and wife crew to sail around the world more than once. Their logs and maps make fascinating reading, and from them Eric wrote and published eleven books. In 1985 they were each awarded the MBE for services to yachting, having 'contributed so much to ocean sailing lore'.

When first married they had a home in Yarmouth, Isle of Wight, but sailed to New Zealand in 1967/8 to live permanently afloat in the Bay of Islands. When Eric died in 1986, Susan sold *Wanderer IV* and returned to live again in Yarmouth. There she led an active life – most importantly she kept sailing. She got to know the local lifeboat crew and got involved with the local RNLI branch, helping to raise funds in the shop.

Maybe it was then that she decided to mark the wonderful life she and her husband had enjoyed afloat by providing the RNLI with a lifeboat. When she died in 1995, just before her eightieth birthday, it was agreed with her family that there could be no better place for that lifeboat than Yarmouth, even though it would be four years before the current lifeboat was scheduled for replacement. At the same time, another matter was agreed between her family and the RNLI: the lifeboat would be named *Eric and Susan Hiscock (Wanderer)*, as a way of ensuring a fitting memorial for these outstanding – and generous – sailors.

I'd like to make a donation …

The earliest money the RNLI received came in the form of subscriptions and individual gifts. People have continued to subscribe to the various membership schemes and this remains a significant source of income. Individual major gifts are frequently used to fund major capital expenditures such as lifeboats and boathouses. Often these donors are women, and because there have been so many over the years it is impossible to include them all. Here are some of the more recent, who have either agreed personally to involvement in this book, or whose family has allowed their story to be told.

Yolande Rampton

Yolande was an only child, but had a large number of cousins – twenty-eight in fact. She was the eldest, and it was because of this position in her family that she first became involved with the RNLI.

Late in life her aunt, Miss Hetty Rampton, took a special interest in Yolande who was by now an adult, still living at home and working in London. When Hetty died she made generous provision for this niece in her will, but also left a sizeable legacy to the RNLI. It was sufficient to secure the naming rights for an all-weather lifeboat. The lifeboat station destined to receive *Hetty Rampton* was Porthdinllaen in North Wales.

Yolande had never been to Porthdinllaen before, but when she was asked if she would name her aunt's lifeboat, she immediately felt it to be an honour and a privilege – even if she felt daunted at the prospect! Firstly, she needed to solve the question of how to get there, and help with this was given by another cousin, Mrs Mildred Baird, who willingly offered to be her chauffeur.

The anxieties Yolande felt about this big event were short-lived, as her welcome at Porthdinllaen was so warm and friendly. Yolande and Mildred were immediately impressed by such kindness but, more importantly, by what the lifeboat crew did. It was a revelation and one that was not to be forgotten for the rest of Yolande's life.

She was very motivated to donate some of her own inheritance from her aunt and organised to do so, funding a D class lifeboat for Hastings Lifeboat Station and naming it in memory of her mother, *Cecile Rampton*. Now Yolande had associations with two lifeboat stations and she eagerly followed the work of both lifeboats. She thoroughly enjoyed the special relationships forged there and started to make regular gifts to support the wider work of the RNLI, as well as making provision in her will.

When the RNLI was looking for an individual to feature in a legacy marketing video, Yolande was an obvious choice and she agreed to the request willingly. It involved being filmed walking across the beach at Hastings talking about the great value of the lifesaving work of the RNLI and why she personally supported the cause. For a lady who now needed to walk with the aid of a stick, the uneven shingle beach, combined with wild weather, were not the easiest for her to manage while clearly saying 'her piece'. But Yolande was undaunted. In her mind she was doing her bit for the crews, and as she looked out to sea at the *Cecile Rampton* bouncing through the waves, her heart was clearly on her sleeve as, unscripted, she said, 'I like that little boat'.

Understanding that the men and women volunteering to be lifeboat crew were unlikely to have a maritime background and so needed thorough training from the RNLI, she responded promptly when a fundraising campaign to support Crew Training was launched in 1995. The campaign was led by two resourceful ladies, Lady Poppy Cooksey and Rosalie Trinder, and ultimately raised £1 million. Yolande personally gave generous donations to support training programmes at Porthdinllaen and Hastings Lifeboat Stations. The people who risked their lives on lifeboats carrying the name *Rampton* meant much to her – and it was not long before it was made clear that she meant much to them, too.

When Yolande learned that the service life of *Cecile Rampton* would end in 1998, she told the RNLI that she wanted to fund the replacement lifeboat and name her *Cecile Rampton II*. This news was greeted with great enthusiasm at Hastings and the station looked forward to welcoming their donor to the naming ceremony, as had happened formerly. Sadly, because Yolande's health had deteriorated, she said that with great regret she would not be able to travel to Hastings. The reaction from the lifeboat station was immediate: 'If Yolande cannot come to the lifeboat, we shall take the lifeboat to her!' They were determined to find a way

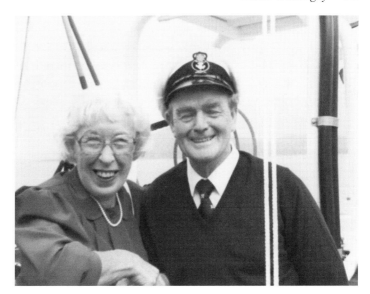

Yolande Rampton with
Coxswain Griffiths Jones,
Porthdinllaen, in 1987
after she had named the
lifeboat *Hetty Rampton*.

to make it possible for her to name the lifeboat. And so it was that a relief D class lifeboat was placed on service at Hastings and *Cecile Rampton II* was placed on a trailer. A coach was hired and over fifty people – crew, committee and ladies' guild – made their way to a car park on the Epsom Downs where the scene was set for one of the most unusual lifeboat namings ever. The 'Mountain had come to Mohammed', and Yolande, overwhelmed by such affection and support, named the lifeboat with not a drop of sea water in sight!

Yolande Rampton was never very concerned to spend money on herself; she preferred to use it to help others. The National Trust and local hospital were causes she supported, as well as the RNLI. At her funeral in 2008, her family reflected on what her involvement with the cause of lifesaving had meant to such a quiet person whose main interests were art and gardening. 'I think she felt that she mattered, whereas before she felt a nobody. She really felt she was perhaps making a difference,' concludes her cousin Mildred Baird.

Mildred too has been keenly affected by her contact with the RNLI, and made an important contribution to Hastings Lifeboat Station when she funded an all-terrain vehicle to enable launch and recovery of *Cecile Rampton II* across the shingle beach – yet more evidence of the power of family values in the RNLI.

Phyl Cleare

'I'll go on forever – you'll be sorry you ever mentioned it!' Phyl Cleare laughs as she describes what she says to people who ask about 'her' lifeboats. A lady with a sharp sense of humour, she knows herself well and is all too aware that her enthusiasm for the RNLI can start her on a long explanation of why the charity deserves support.

'I always encourage everyone to give,' she says, and then recalls how, when she made her first transatlantic crossing on the *Queen Mary 2* and discovered there was no RNLI collecting box, she was resolved to do something about it. 'I spoke to the Purser and told him that there was always a box on the *Queen Elizabeth 2* and that he should contact RNLI Headquarters to get one – and tell them I sent you!' She was not too sure that he took very well to these instructions: 'He seemed to have a lot of excuses, but on my next voyage I went looking for the RNLI box – and sure enough, there was one there. Good thing too!'

When asked, Phyl will answer that she cannot remember why it was that she first chose to support the RNLI with the gift of a lifeboat in 1990. 'Maybe it was because I don't fly and so any overseas travel is always by ship – but I'm not sure.' What is sure is that Phyl and her husband Jack, who have always been active travellers, became deeply committed to the RNLI after that.

Phyl lives in an apartment in Bournemouth, whose walls are covered with pictures of all four lifeboats she has given, and she has numerous photograph albums and news cuttings. They include two D class lifeboats both stationed at Swanage – *Phyl Clare* and *Phyl Clare 2* – and the Atlantic 75, *Phyl Clare 3*, stationed at Weymouth. The fourth lifeboat, the Swanage D class *Jack Cleare*, was given in memory of her husband who died in 2001. This is quite a fleet of lifeboats, but Phyl has clearly not finished yet, having made provision for a *Jack Cleare 2* at Swanage when the time comes, as well as a legacy which she hopes will enable the provision of a lifeboat to carry both their names: *Jack and Phyl Cleare*.

It is very obvious that her engagement with the RNLI does not stop with having provided the lifeboats, because Phyl cares so passionately about the crews. Living close to the sea, she keeps a close eye on the conditions: 'If it is rough, I ring up the Swanage and Weymouth Lifeboat Stations and ask what has happened. I think these people are remarkable, but I do worry about them.' Not only does she think about the crews out at sea, she is concerned about the families waiting at home for them to return. Her awareness of their feelings dates back to a conversation she once had with a crew member after he had been awarded a gallantry medal. She asked him what his wife had thought that night, and when she received the answer, 'I think she just turned over and went back to sleep', she had her doubts. Later she spoke to his wife, repeating what her husband had said. 'It wasn't quite like that,' said the wife. Phyl has never forgotten the understated courage and dignity of that woman and makes a point of acknowledging the bravery of the families in her speech at the naming of a lifeboat.

A strong bond of friendship has grown between Phyl and the two lifeboat stations in Dorset. It is one of mutual respect and affection – and great generosity. Phyl likes to be sure that neither crew goes thirsty at Christmas! Her interest in the workings of the RNLI means that she visits Headquarters, the Lifeboat College and Open Days regularly. She likes to be kept in the picture about any new developments. She recalls one time when she went to Poole on the occasion of an official visit from HRH the Duke of Kent:

> I had been told that his time was limited and please not to initiate a conversation with him – only speak if spoken to! When he reached me I showed him a picture of my two boats. He took it in his hands but then realised he needed his spectacles. With great care he took the case out of his pocket, opened it and put them on. It seemed to take forever and I thought I would be in trouble for delaying him. But no, he looked very closely and asked me some questions before thanking me for bringing them and only then he moved on. I thought he was so kind.

Even after all these years of such close relationship with the RNLI, Phyl has never been afloat on a lifeboat: 'You will never catch me doing that,' she says, 'but I'll talk to anyone

Phyl Cleare naming the Swanage D class lifeboat *Jack Cleare* in August 2003.

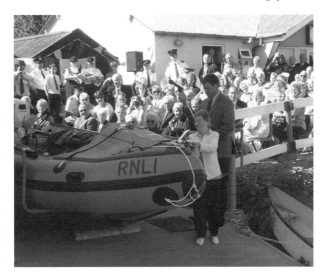

about how wonderful lifeboats and their crews are and then I'll tell them that they should give money to the RNLI.'

In recognition of such exceptional commitment to the cause of saving life at sea, Phyl Cleare was awarded the Southwest Region RNLI Supporter of the Year in 2005.

Georgina Taylor

The family values that lie at the heart of all lifeboat crews and communities are readily rec-ognised by virtually everyone entering any of the stations around the coast. Major donors frequently develop a very special relationship with their station and some, like Georgina Taylor, become an integral part of the family.

Georgina was every inch a country woman; she was born on a farm in Bedfordshire and joined the Women's Land Army in 1939. In 1945 she toyed with the idea of going to the Falklands Islands, whose men were advertising for wives, but on reflection decided that the Scilly Isles were a better bet. Her job there was to run the cattle on Tresco. It was a fortunate choice because the Land Agent, Stanley Taylor, was an eligible bachelor who she fell in love with and married. It was this experience of island life that introduced her to the work of the RNLI. Georgina saw how important St Mary's lifeboat was, both for the residents and also for those on passage near these scattered islands. The lifesaving work of St Mary's lifeboat crew made a powerful impression on her, and one which would influence her greatly in later life.

The Taylors moved to farm in Wiltshire for a number of years and retired to Pewsey, where gardening became the focus of their attention. When Stanley died, Georgina decided that a lifeboat was better than a headstone. Her approach to the RNLI revealed that inshore lifeboats were scheduled for replacement at Tenby and New Brighton. Not knowing either place, she decided to investigate and chose to visit Tenby first.

Arthur Squibbs, who was then Station Honorary Secretary, remembers the day:

Georgina came to Tenby on a still, sunny and warm day. She was shown around the boathouse, leaving the Harbour by way of the Dead House Steps – so called because the town mortu-ary used to be sited half way up. When seated overlooking the bay and fortified with a cup of tea she said, 'I was assured the site was flat!' We all held our breath but all was well and it soon became obvious that she would look no further for a home for Stanley's lifeboat, such was her enthusiasm for Tenby.

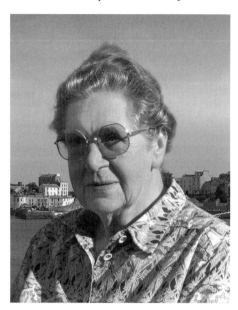

Georgina Taylor on one of her visits to Tenby.

After the lifeboat entered service, Georgina made regular visits to Tenby – usually four times a year, and mainly on anniversaries when she would be left alone for as long as she wished in the boathouse with her memories. Arthur was placed in a difficult position when, on an early visit, she expressed a wish to go afloat in 'her' boat. 'This was against the rules, but the station mechanic, supported by crew, took her to sea.' Arthur waited anxiously for their return: 'I was concerned about the consequences if something had gone wrong, but all was well – they had been seal watching!' This was a happy experience Georgina often spoke of.

She was anything but a demanding person, although her appearance in Tenby Harbour has been described as akin to a 'Royal Progress' because crew appeared from nowhere anxious to ply her with tea and cakes. Blessed with a good memory for names and having a genuine interest in them and their lives, she sat on the wall and chatted easily for hours. In fact, Georgina was bonding with her new family. Once she said to me: 'You see, Sue, I thought that because we had no children I would have no one when Stanley died. I was wrong; Tenby Lifeboat Station is my family.' She made this statement as she handed me a cheque to fund the successor to the *Stanley Taylor* when it was ready for replacement. As powerful a statement of her support and commitment for Tenby as is possible to make.

Like a benevolent senior member of the family, Georgina decided that she wanted to give a different sort of help to the younger members of the crew – help that would make something possible for them which would otherwise be unaffordable. She had in mind to sponsor an individual on a Tall Ships voyage with the Sail Training Association. This was such great generosity and a wonderful opportunity for someone, but how was that individual to be selected? Eventually it was resolved by the random chance of matching the Lottery Bonus Ball with a crew number. The lucky young man went on the voyage of a lifetime that changed his life. He believes that the experience he had helped him mature from a rather wild youth into a responsible citizen. Georgina was delighted and made provision for others to follow in subsequent years. She did it not for any thanks or favour, but because these young men were, in her heart, her family.

When she died in 2005, her lifeboat family was there in numbers to carry her coffin and to join with other family and friends to say farewell to a special lady. One of the pallbearers had one further task to perform for her – to scatter her ashes from 'her' boat following the memorial service in St Julian's Fisherman's Chapel. Yes, it was the first recipient of the Tall Ships voyage!

Her name lives on in Tenby – her third gift of a lifeboat, *Georgina Stanley Taylor*, was funded from her legacy to the RNLI and entered service in December 2009.

Postscript

While living on Tresco, Georgina made a lasting friendship with a young teacher, Anita Greenwood. Anita, too, loved the sea and so was very interested in Georgina's involvement with the RNLI. She happily accepted an invitation to the naming ceremony at Tenby and was very impressed with the commitment of everyone in the lifeboat community. The seed of an idea was planted that day – Anita began to think about giving a lifeboat herself. She discussed it with her friend, Pam Waugh, who thought it such a good idea that she wanted to get involved too.

Rusper is the name of the inshore lifeboat at Rock Lifeboat Station, Cornwall. It is the name of the village where Anita and Pam live. As with Georgina, who inspired their gift, they hope to increase awareness of the RNLI in their community.

Jane Turnbull

As an avid newspaper reader, Jane Turnbull's attention was caught by a piece in *The Times* describing the work of Humber Lifeboat Station – the only station in the RNLI with a paid crew, since its remote location at the far end of Spurn Point makes volunteering impossible. She read about the Humber Lifeboat Superintendent Coxswain, Brian Bevan, learning that he had been awarded three Gold Medals for gallantry. Next she came to a description of the new Severn class lifeboat that was being built to replace the ageing lifeboat currently in service. Finally, she reached the real point of the article, which was an appeal for money to help fund this new lifeboat.

She had read the piece with growing interest because she had only just received an unexpected financial windfall and thought this might be the perfect way to use the money in a constructive way. She and her husband Bob were not sailors or particularly 'seaside' people and had no previous contact with the RNLI, but this appeal had fired Jane's imagination and she wanted to know more.

Her initial contact with the RNLI team leading the appeal convinced her that she would make the donation, and it was not long before she and Bob received an invitation to attend the self-righting trial of the lifeboat. It was a memorable moment, Jane says: 'I remember seeing her being hauled upside down and then watching her shaking water off herself – an amazing sight!' It was then that Jane and Bob realised just how sophisticated is the engineering of a modern lifeboat, and they were hungry to learn more. Meeting Brian Bevan that day was further proof that she had entered a world of very special people. Thirteen years later, and having since met many more men and women lifeboat crew members, Jane

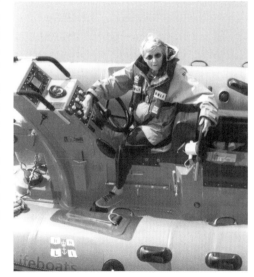

Jane Turnbull taking a close look at *Bob Turnbull* while visiting Ramsgate Lifeboat Station in 2010.

reflects: 'They are a race apart.' This admiration constantly sustains her motivation to continue her support for their lifesaving work.

When Bob died in 1998, he left money to the RNLI and Jane hoped that it might be possible to fund a lifeboat to carry his name. It was, and the name *Bob Turnbull* is to be seen on the Atlantic 75 stationed at Ramsgate. Jane named the lifeboat herself – a very happy and moving occasion for her.

Not only does she like to visit Ramsgate and learn about the work of the station and crew, she likes to update her knowledge of the wider organisation, and visiting Poole Headquarters periodically enables her to learn what developments are being planned. A visit in September 2009 brought a great surprise – the chance to go afloat on a Tamar class lifeboat. Even better, to steer her. Not normally known for a lack of words in any situation, Jane was virtually speechless afterwards!

She is, however, very articulate about the benefits she sees in giving support to the RNLI: 'They are immeasurable. If the Government – of any shade – had anything to do with it, it would be a monumental shambles and a waste.'

Betty Battle

Some very special relationships develop between donors and lifeboat stations. It is always for the donor to choose how much or how little contact they wish to have, but sometimes the chemistry just works!

A very active and successful RNLI Branch fundraiser, Betty became closely involved with Hayling Island Lifeboat Station. Lifeboat Operations Manager, Nigel Roper, explains:

> If I recall correctly, my first conversation with Betty Battle was in early 1994 when she told me that she and her husband Derrick had funded an Atlantic 75 and that she understood from RNLI Headquarters that the Atlantic was to be stationed at Hayling Island on the South Coast and I was asked 'Where is Hayling Island'? I told her we were just east of Portsmouth on the Hampshire / West Sussex border and at the entrance to Chichester Harbour.
>
> Betty explained that Derrick had funded a Scholarship at a New Zealand University and that he would make available a similar for her 'to do with as she pleased'. Betty, already the Chair of the RNLI Ashtead Fundraising Branch, knew immediately that she wanted to buy a lifeboat. Even at that early stage, Derrick and particularly Betty were thrilled at the prospect of 'her lifeboat' being stationed on the nearest part of the coast to their home in Ashtead. I went on to outline that our station had recently been demolished but that I would be delighted to meet up with them. I explained that the proposed new station being built would not only house a B Class lifeboat but also a D Class lifeboat.

All arrangements moved smoothly forward, including the naming ceremony at which Betty duly named the lifeboat *Betty Battle*. A bond had been established, and in no time Betty and her husband were keen to visit again, quite innocently giving Nigel Roper something of a dilemma. He recalls:

> On one of their first visits to the rebuilt station, Betty and Derrick asked to be taken out in the Harbour in 'their lifeboat'. Under benign conditions I have to say (and strictly against

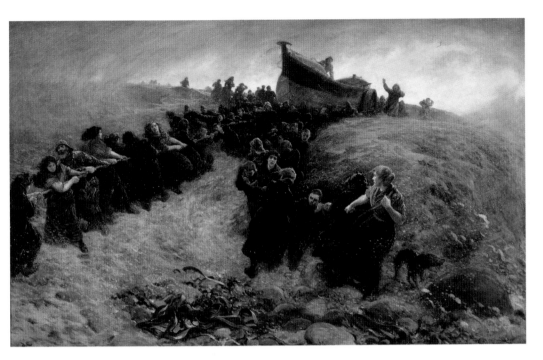

1 'The Women': a painting by John Charlton depicting women launching the Cullercoats lifeboat to the rescue of *Lovely Nelly* in 1861. (The Laing Gallery, Newcastle)

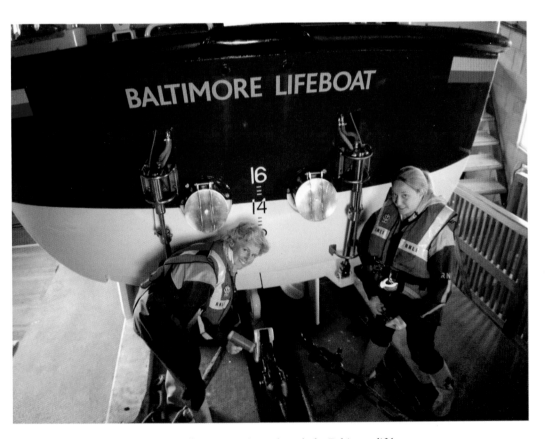

2 Rianne Smith and Kate Callanan preparing to launch the Baltimore lifeboat.

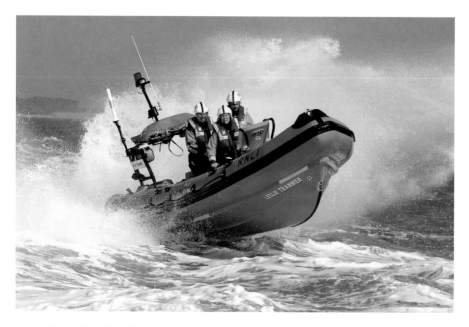

3 Cath Fox of Southwold at the helm of the Atlantic 75 lifeboat *Leslie Tranmer*.

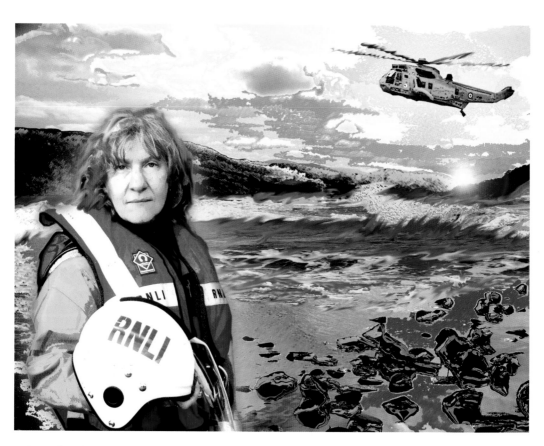

4 *Partnership* – a digital image of Vivian Bailey. One of a series created for Lock Ness Lifeboat Station by David Evans Bailey.

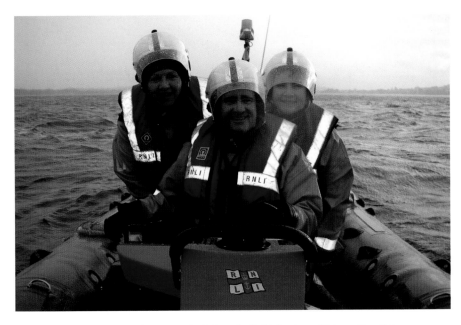

5 Eleanor Hooker of Lough Derg at the helm of relief Atlantic 75 lifeboat *Vera Skilton*.

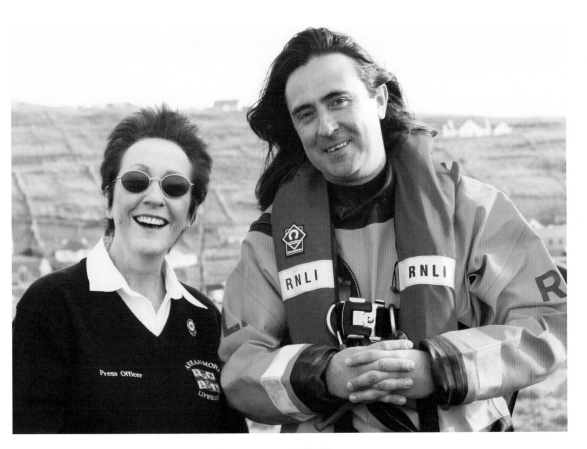

6 Nora Flanangan of Arranmore with TV presenter Neil Oliver.

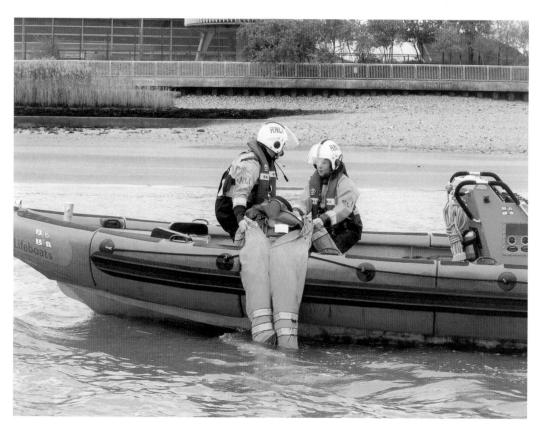

7 Sue Body of Tower Lifeboat Station on a training exercise with fellow crew member Robin Jenkins.

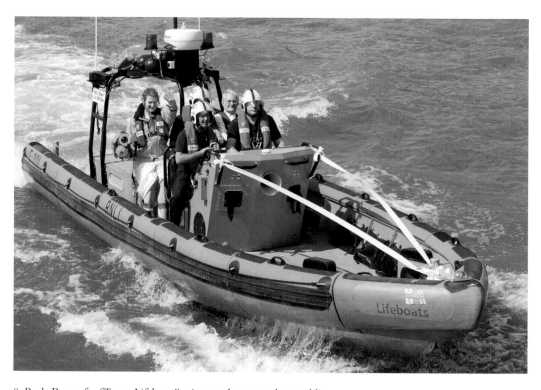

8 Paula Bancroft of Tower Lifeboat Station on the way to her wedding.

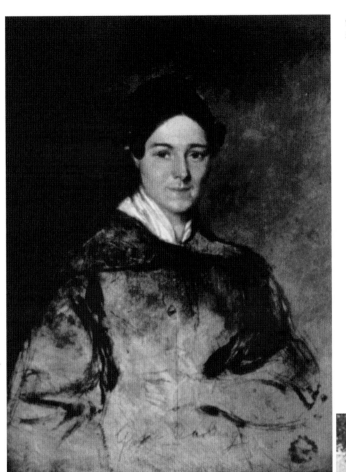

9 Grace Darling – the first woman to be awarded an RNLI medal for bravery.

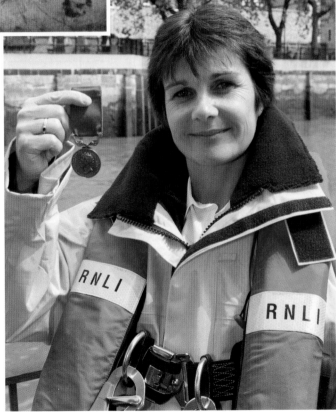

10 Aileen Jones of Porthcawl – in 2004 the first female crew member to be awarded the RNLI Silver Medal for Gallantry.

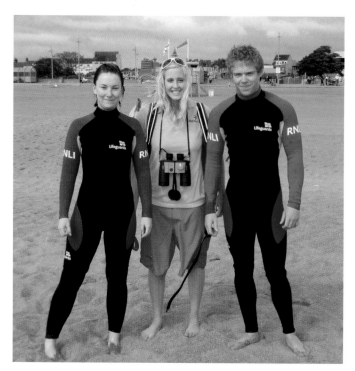

11 Kelly Blackburn (left) on the day the RNLI Lifeguard service was launched in East Lindsey.

12 A postcard perspective of the women who waited for the safe return of their loved ones. (Iain Booth postcard collection)

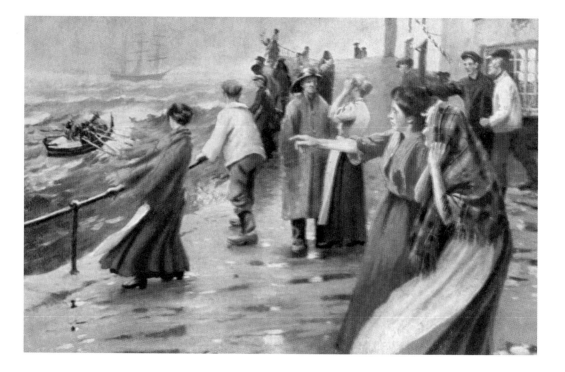

Opposite from top

13 The Duchess of Kent on board the Workington lifeboat *Sir John Fisher* during a visit to Cumbria in 1995.

14 The Ceremony of Dedication of the RNLI Memorial in Poole, Dorset on 3 September 2009. Crew representatives of each operational division read out the 778 names of the lost. Left to right: Gary Gibbs (south), Dave Steenvoorden (north), Kenny Peters (Scotland), Peter Huxtable (east), Billy Scully (Ireland), Roy Griffiths (Wales and west). (RNLI/Nigel Mallard)

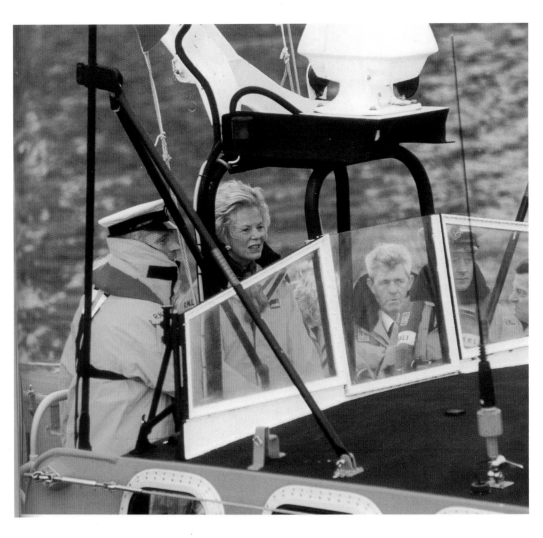

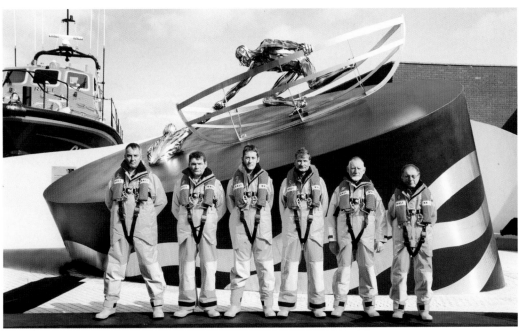

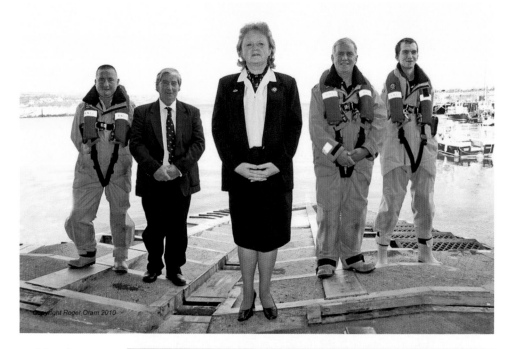

15 Mary Corran, Lifeboat Operations Manager at Douglas Lifeboat Station, with (left to right) son Brendan, husband Robert, brother-in-law Neil and nephew Ryan – all Corrans!

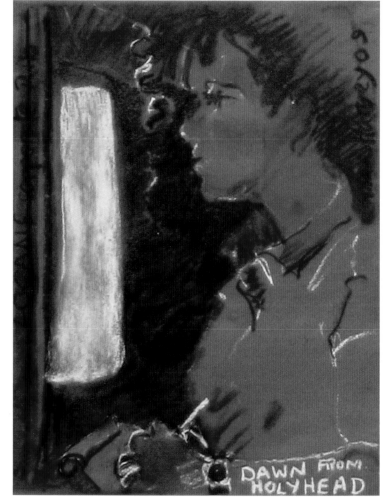

DAWN FROM. HOLYHEAD

16 'She Who Would Valiant Be' – a woman crew member from Holyhead depicted by artist Minna Harvey for an exhibition at the Lifeboat College on training RNLI volunteers.

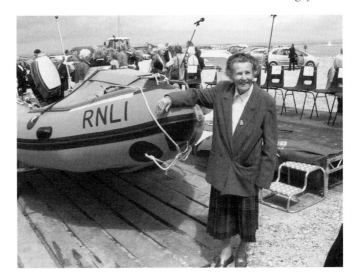

Betty Battle at the naming ceremony for the inshore lifeboat *Amanda, James and Ben* at Hayling Island in 2005 – funded by her and named after her grandchildren.

regulations!) I somewhat reluctantly agreed as to refuse I felt would cause some difficulty and embarrassment. Needless to say, squeezing Betty into a dry suit brought about much humour! Fortunately for all concerned, they enjoyed their voyage *up harbour* which went without mishap.

A couple of years later Derrick Battle died, but Betty continued her visits to Hayling Island, making it her business to get to know the individual crew members and, with Nigel's help, taking home an enlargement of the bi-annual crew photo with each member of the station identified. She took an active interest in all the shouts – she just loved the fact that 'her lifeboat' was out there doing what she was designed for and saving lives. Betty became very much part of the RNLI family at Hayling Island, usually driving down on a Sunday as she knew that it was the day for all to gather at the station to carry out boat checks, etc. She would be kind enough to bring cakes with her, and Nigel relates with amusement:

> I think Betty would be the first to admit that cooking was not her particular interest or passion and her fruit cakes resembled bricks, both in shape and texture! Good ballast! Nevertheless, always consumed with relish.

Betty wanted to give even more support to Hayling Island Lifeboat Station, and on discovering that the D class was scheduled for replacement, she agreed to start the process of funding a new D Class lifeboat. It transpired that this lifeboat was to be the new version of the D class, and was to be rather more expensive. This did not deter her – which is particularly poignant, as by now she was suffering from cancer of the spine. In May 2005, the lifeboat was delivered on the Thursday and named the following Saturday to ensure that Betty was well enough to complete the naming ceremony. She named the lifeboat *Amanda, James & Ben* after her grandchildren.

Sadly Betty died in November 2006. Because of her long association with the station and the high regard that Betty was held in by the helmsman and crews, they went up to Ashtead from the coast to act as pallbearers. Nigel recalls the funeral:

The weather was poor with heavy rain but just as the coffin was about to be carried in, the sun came out right on cue. It was announced from the altar at her funeral that she had in fact completed funding of the new B Class Lifeboat Atlantic 85 B-829 and this was to be named after her late husband Derrick.

In February of 2009, B-829 *Derrick Battle* arrived on station at Hayling Island.

This very generous and unassuming lady has made possible three lifeboats for Hayling Island, and in recognition of that and of their great affection for her, the station has named their tractor *Betty* in her honour. As Nigel Roper explains:

> This is the purpose-built 4 x 4 tractor used to launch the B Class lifeboat so in a sense, we have kept the family together and helps us to explain to our visitors, the story of the unqualified support of both Betty and Derrick, neither of whom used to sail!

Evelyn Paley

A holiday in Padstow at the age of eight, which included a visit to the lifeboat station, proved to be a powerful experience for Evelyn Paley, and one which gave her a fascination with the RNLI that she would carry all her life. It was the sight of the lifeboat that so impressed her. She says:

> I was used to messing about in boats on the River Thames where we lived, but this lifeboat was a rowing boat – it was beyond my comprehension and I just could not believe it! How anyone could manipulate it was quite amazing to me as a child. Ever since then I have been interested in the RNLI and have attended lectures and demonstrations, which has kept the spirit alive.

Evelyn married a surgeon who was also a keen sailor. When he died in 1995, she thought about the right way to remember him and readily decided that a lifeboat to carry his name was the solution. This would also have the additional benefit of keeping alive their mutual interest in the RNLI.

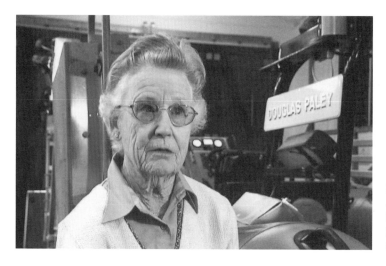

Evelyn Paley at Appledore Lifeboat Station while filming a legacy marketing video for the RNLI.

On the north coast of Devon at Appledore Lifeboat Station, the Atlantic 75 lifeboat carries the name *Douglas Paley*. The crew are proud for their lifeboat to carry this name, having been told by Evelyn when she named the lifeboat that her husband had worked at East Grinstead Hospital during and after the Second World War with Sir Archibald McIndoe, healing and reconstructing the faces of airmen who were burned and badly injured when shot down by the enemy.

It is a happy relationship that has grown between Evelyn and Appledore Lifeboat Station. Avidly she reads reports of the work of the lifeboat and usually visits once a year to learn first-hand about how crew and lifeboat have functioned together to save life. 'I am welcomed with great enthusiasm,' she says, 'and my admiration for them knows no bounds.' She was more than pleased to tell this to the world when asked by the RNLI in 2006 if she would feature in a legacy marketing video. 'I was very happy to help in encouraging people to leave a legacy to the RNLI, as of course I have done.'

Sally Anne Odell

'Unless you've travelled on the sea, you don't realise how wicked the sea is,' observes Sally Odell, who has been cruising on the sea since the 1950s. She follows a firm family tradition – her Great Aunt Kate was a photographer with a well-established practice of going on all maiden voyages. Yes, she was on the *Titanic*, and on Sally's sitting room wall there is a photograph to prove it. Sally's father was also bitten by the cruising bug. An entrepreneur with business interests in many different countries, he rejected air travel in preference for visiting his companies by ship. So when Sally learned of her inheritance when her father died in 1997 and financial advisors floated the idea of making gifts to charities, it is hardly surprising that one of the charities she thought of was the RNLI:

> It wasn't just my love of cruising, it was tied in with the TV programme *Blue Peter*. I loved it and collected for them with a passion – I raided both our house and the neighbours - probably made myself very unpopular! It was when I was watching the *Blue Peter* presenters showing the lifeboats we were collecting for that I said to my Mother, one day I'm going to have a lifeboat with my name on it – I'll leave some money in my will for it. My mother wasn't encouraging: 'Well, you won't see it will you, you'll be dead!'

Sally Odell, very much alive and full of fun, has certainly seen her name on a lifeboat – it is an Atlantic 75 stationed at Kinsale in the Republic of Ireland. The name on the lifeboat is *Miss Sally Anne (Baggy)*.

Sally took the opportunity of her handover speech at the naming ceremony in November 2003 to explain the inclusion of the word 'Baggy'. In 1997 she was diagnosed with bowel cancer. After trying an experimental non-invasive treatment recommended by her consultant, she eventually had to have a colostomy. Sally's love of life and her determination to make the most of everything is matched by a very wicked sense of humour – hence the word 'Baggy' in the lifeboat name – but her aim is also to encourage others, she says. It got a clap and a big cheer from everyone attending the ceremony.

Since then, her medical journey has been fraught with many serious complications and much pain, but Sally has had an amazingly varied life from working as a hospital welfare officer in Germany and Cyprus to working as a deputy sheriff in Wyoming (yes, keys to the jail and all), and she continues to look for and celebrate the good things in life. She admits that she had no idea at all how powerful the experience of providing a lifeboat would be: 'It doesn't come home to roost until you see the boat on the water. I don't have children of my own, but it must be like seeing your child in a nativity play.'

Her first sight of *Miss Sally Anne (Baggy)* on the water was from on board the cruise ship *Artemis* when the crew brought the lifeboat out to the ship to greet its donor while she was cruising off the coast of County Cork:

> I was so excited and just shouted out *there's my boys* – the other passengers were intrigued, so I explained why they should support the RNLI. People have a tendency to take the service provided by the RNLI for granted. They think they are just *there* and will automatically come out to rescue them.

Sally Odell describes a range of experiences she has had with charities, and is quick to point out that many make the two big mistakes that most alienate her. Forgetting to say thank you is the first, which she considers unforgivable. The other misjudgement is to invite her to what Sally terms 'posh dos'. This is not what she wants her donations to be spent on, and she believes it to be a misuse of charitable money. Charities making these errors are swiftly dropped. By contrast, the relationship with Kinsale Lifeboat Station means so much to Sally that when she learned of the plans to build a boathouse, she quickly volunteered a generous donation to kick-start the fund. Her links with the Personal Donations Department are important, too: 'I enjoy their enthusiasm but value their serenity – I have positive conversations about my support for the RNLI.'

Her engagement with 'my boys' grows stronger, and she is looking forward to seeing them when she takes another cruise to Ireland in 2010. Her zest for life is infectious, as is her enthusiasm for the Kinsale lifeboat: 'People may get a bit sick of hearing about my boat … tough!'

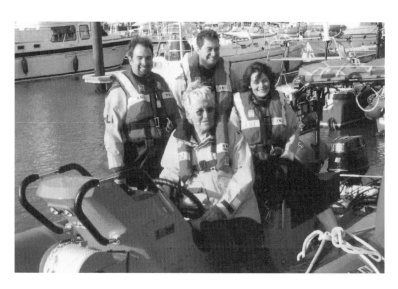

Sally Anne Odell at Cowes, Isle of Wight in 2003 for the naming of the Atlantic 75 lifeboat she had provided for Kinsale Lifeboat Station.

Kay Hurley MBE

Reading about the plans being made by the RNLI to establish a lifeboat service on the River Thames stirred Yorkshire childhood memories for Mrs Kay Hurley. She recalled what she thought to be 'magic', when there was a disaster at sea and the lifeboat crews seemed to appear out of nowhere, save people, and then disappear again. Well, as a small girl living on a farm miles from the sea, this is how it seemed to her, thanks to what was reported in the *Yorkshire Post*.

As a person with an acute understanding of the power of the River Thames and feeling much sadness for the young people who had lost their lives on the night of the *Marchioness* disaster, she thought she would like to provide the funds for one of the new lifeboats to be stationed on the River Thames. She knew that her Australian husband would have approved of this, as he was a keen oarsman.

She was disappointed to discover that all of the first generation of lifeboats had already been funded, but listened carefully when told about another significant operational development, which was the deployment of hovercraft at some lifeboat stations. These were locations on muddy and sandy estuaries where conditions often made it difficult for inshore lifeboats to operate effectively. A hovercraft, which 'flies' over the mud, sandbanks and shallow water, could well make the difference between life and death when trying to reach a casualty in such conditions. The RNLI had been actively exploring the concept and trialling a prototype craft to establish the viability of introducing a limited number of hovercraft at relevant locations.

'Being a Yorkshire woman, I wanted to know where my money was going, so I went to see for myself what was being described to me,' Kay recalled. 'I was amazed; it was the first hovercraft I had ever seen and all the equipment impressed me greatly.' She quickly made her decision, 'Yes, I will do that' – but she had another request: 'Will I be able to fly her?' With the imminent prospect of securing the money to build the first operational RNLI hovercraft, the answer came back, 'Yes!' And so it was that the diminutive Kay Hurley donned the mandatory personal protection kit and, with the guidance of Tony Stankus, RNLI Hovercraft Development Manager, flew the hovercraft across Holes Bay in Poole Harbour. 'It was fascinating – a real adventure for an elderly lady,' she says as a smile fills her face.

She learned that the hovercraft was to be stationed at Morecambe in Lancashire, a place with a combination of quicksand, mud and dangerous fast rising tides that are second to none. Her next task was to choose its name in readiness for the naming ceremony that would take place after the hovercraft had entered service in December 2002. In recognition of its great speed and modus operandi, the name she chose for H-002 was *The Hurley Flyer*.

And how fortunate it was that this flying machine was in the hands of competent RNLI lifesavers on the night of 5 February 2004! This small craft, along with the Morecambe Lifeboat Station inshore and all-weather lifeboats, helicopters, coastguard teams and private rescue services, went to the aid of over thirty Chinese cocklers caught in the powerful incoming tide as they worked under cover of darkness to gather cockles. Their illegal, profit-seeking gangmasters had paid insufficient heed to the notorious dangers of Morecambe Bay, putting their countrymen in mortal danger. The men had no safety gear and some were plucked from the sea naked because, in their desperation to swim to safety, they had taken off their clothes.

Miles away in the safety of her home, Kay Hurley watched reports on the television news but it was not long before she was contacted by RNLI volunteers at Morecambe to tell her personally what had happened and how *The Hurley Flyer* had played such a significant role in the rescue. She recalls her feelings at the time:

> I agonised for the poor victims who had been abused by the gangmasters, but was anxious for the crew. I am always concerned because they leave at the drop of a hat, running and often putting on their kit as they go. But they have an invisible bond – they have to have this because of the danger they face. Their camaraderie is exceptional.

Kay, who was a teacher with a wide experience in challenging schools worldwide, says: 'I have dealt with young men in various countries of the world but I have *never* met young men like those in the RNLI!'

This Yorkshire woman's instinct for spending money well inspired her decision to provide the funds for H-005 which was to be stationed at New Brighton, on Merseyside. Her taste for 'getting involved' was again fulfilled when she accompanied the delivery of a launching trailer for the hovercraft from Poole to New Brighton:

> I sat in the cabin of our vehicle as we made our way up the motorway, feeling like a queen as other truck drivers saluted the RNLI lorry as we made our way north – that says a lot about what the public think of the RNLI.

In her desire to feel a part of the station community, Kay visited New Brighton a few times before the official naming of the *Hurley Spirit* in 2005. The real bond this created between donor and station is revealed in Kay's most recent visit to Merseyside in 2009. Delighting

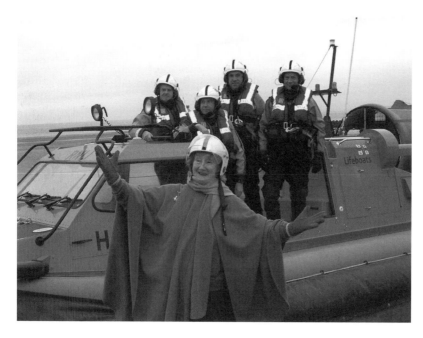

Kay Hurley. with *The Hurley Flyer* and crew at Morecambe at the naming ceremony in 2003.

all by arriving in a helicopter and then standing everyone a fish and chip lunch, she was greeted by Station President, Frank Brereton, with the words: 'Welcome, esteemed guest'. Kay responded, 'Please don't say that, call me one of the family'.

History has a curious way of going in circles, and this is just what has happened for this particular 'woman of the RNLI'. Having done great service on the busy River Thames, there is now a need to replace the first generation of lifeboats operating on the river ... and yes, Mrs Hurley has already agreed to provide funds for one of these E class lifeboats.

Anne Bache

Anne was very keen to accept the invitation for the ceremony at which the inshore lifeboat her brother and sister-in-law had donated to Burry Port was to be named by their four grandchildren. She had been a keen sailor for many years and understood the importance of the lifeboat service. It was, though, her first insight into the operation of a lifeboat station and she was impressed. She also saw the pleasure her brother and sister-in-law had in giving a lifeboat and said: 'This is rather fun. How do you go about it?'

Anne first sailed at the Midlands Sailing Club at Edgbaston Reservoir, close to the centre of Birmingham. As her enthusiasm grew she and friends chartered and then purchased their own yacht, which was based on the River Fal in Cornwall. She particularly enjoyed these waters and so was quite delighted that her offer to donate an inshore lifeboat was gratefully received, with the proposal by the RNLI that it should be based at Teignmouth.

The lifeboat was still being built, but keen to see where its home would be, she proposed a family trip to meet everyone at Teignmouth Lifeboat Station. A warm welcome awaited them and even though it was apparent to all that Anne was somewhat frail, a trip afloat to see a training exercise was proposed. After donning a dry suit and lifejacket, Anne was taken for a gentle 'potter' around the harbour. Anne pointed to the open sea and said to the crew:

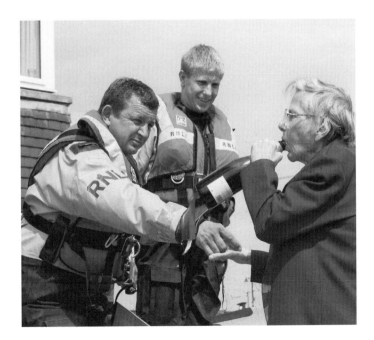

Anne Bache enjoying champagne before preparing to speak at the naming ceremony of *The Two Annes*.

'I thought they went out there.' 'Well yes, but …' came the diplomatic answer. 'Aren't we going out there then?' quizzed Anne. Anne's wishes were granted, and lunch that day was a little later than planned!

Anne had cancer and obviously knew how advanced it was because when she was told the likely date of the naming ceremony for her boat, she replied with, 'In that case, I'm afraid I won't be there'. Fortunately it proved possible to organise an earlier date and Anne was present, by now needing to use a wheelchair. She had decided to name the lifeboat *The Two Annes*, after herself and her sister-in-law, Ann, who unfortunately was in hospital and missed the earlier naming ceremony at Burry Port.

How Anne's great strength of character and determination shine clearly through! Her brother, Bill, confirms that she always was a very competent and single-minded person. They worked together in the family firm, which designed and manufactured pressure gauges and switches. Anne ultimately became the Chairman, but earlier as sales director had a ready answer for any men who, on hearing her voice at the end of the telephone, asked to speak to a man: 'If my degree in physics and maths is not good enough for you, we don't want your business.'

She was very determined to name the lifeboat herself, but was concerned that her throat may be too dry to produce a voice. A glass of water would have served, but when Anne was handed the champagne to pour over the lifeboat, she first put it to her lips and took a quick swig. There were gasps of surprise from all around but it worked and she said the words clearly.

One week later she was admitted to a hospice and five weeks later she died. The bond with Teignmouth had been so strongly forged that seven representatives from the lifeboat

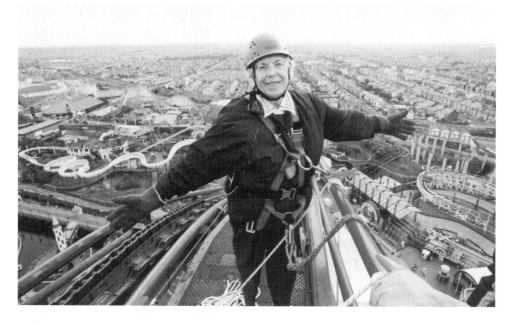

Barbara Page wing-walking on *Utterly Butterly* at the 2003 Blackpool Airshow to raise funds for the RNLI.

station formed a guard of honour at the cremation service. Some weeks later her ashes were scattered from *The Two Annes* at the mouth of the Teign Estuary. At the helm was Jude Chilvers, a woman of whose achievements Anne's brother knows she would have been proud.

I've had this idea …

Barbara Page admits to loving a challenge, so when in 1999 the Townswomen's Guild issued ninety-nine challenges to their members, she picked an exciting one – abseiling. Living in Blackpool, the obvious choice was to abseil from the top of The Big One on the Pleasure Beach. Barbara is also a member of Blackpool Ladies' Lifeboat Guild, and so she spotted an opportunity to raise funds for the RNLI and get some good local publicity.

With £1,500 in the kitty and having had an exhilarating experience, she volunteered for another piece of 'derring do': wing walking on the Utterly Butterly plane at Blackpool Airshow in 2003. With another £1,500 raised for the RNLI, Barbara was very happy but intrigued with the amount of publicity she received for both her ventures and eventually decided that what had fired the media attention was that she was sixty-nine and seventy-three years old at the time.

Chantal Carr

Having a dad who was a passionate supporter of the RNLI meant that Chantal got her first RNLI T-shirt when she was two, and now has more RNLI tea towels than she cares to think about! When her dad became ill and lost all the energy he had always enjoyed, Chantal realised that since having her two boys, she had allowed herself to become overweight and unfit. Spurred on by her dad's encouragement, she lost ten stone in four years, and with the new lease of life this gave her, signed up for the Great South Run in 2007. Her plan was to surprise her dad by doing the run and giving all the sponsorship to the RNLI. Sadly he died before she could do this, but Chantal did the run anyway and raised £700.

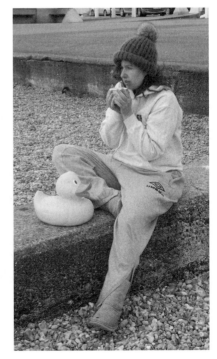

Success tasted sweet and she has done the run again – this time with her son, Tommy, joining her for the mini run, as well as doing the Edinburgh Marathon twice, with all the sponsorship going to the RNLI. Now very firmly involved with the RNLI as an Education Presenter in the London area, Chantal was looking for a really big challenge.

Chantal Carr, who is swimming the English Channel in 2010 to raise funds for the RNLI, warms up after a practice swim at Dover.

The one she has chosen is to swim the Channel. At the time of writing this is scheduled for 14 September 2010. 'I don't think anyone believed me until in May I went down to Dover and took my first dip in the harbour. Ten minutes at about thirteen degrees was enough to make me question what I was doing. During the two-hour drive I decided I had the will-power and I was definitely going back the next day for another shot,' she explains.

What is it that drives her on to put herself through the rigours of the training?

> I am trying to balance the swim and fundraising with the education all the time but it is worth every minute. Nothing is better than enjoying time with the crews at the stations I visit and just the feeling that although I may never have the chance to fulfil my dream to become a crew member, I can hopefully prevent people getting into trouble near the sea

So says the woman who, in wanting to follow her dad's lead, has achieved so much for herself and for the RNLI.

Would it help if …?

Brenda Calderwood

Describing the RNLI as her 'Number 1 Charity', Brenda first became involved in 1965 when a friend in the Ladies' Lifeboat Guild persuaded her to sell raffle tickets at the Seahouses Lifeboat Fête. As so often happens, one thing led to another, and Brenda joined the committee before starting to help at the Seahouses lifeboat shop every weekend. Before very long she was organising the shop and fundraising on Lifeboat Day. As Brenda says, 'I was thoroughly involved!'

Her brother, Derek, shared Brenda's enthusiasm for the RNLI. He was an active member of the Seahouses Lifeboat Station Committee, and for twelve years was the Curator of the Grace Darling Museum in Bamburgh. Since opening in 1938, the museum was run by a

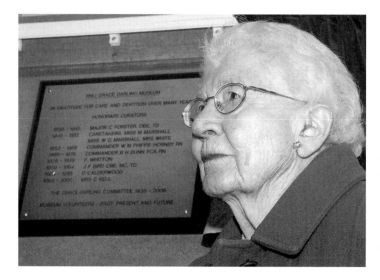

Brenda Calderwood, who unveiled a plaque dedicated to the honorary curators of the Grace Darling Museum, Bamburgh, at the official reopening in 2008. (*Northumberland Gazette*)

committee of local volunteers. Keen to support her brother in the work, Brenda took on the role of secretary and became very active with the work of the group.

All the volunteers worked hard to maintain the museum, which contained many valuable items of national and international significance. However, the building was damp and increasingly it became obvious that professional expertise was needed to ensure the proper conservation of the collection. A national appeal was launched in 2004 with local volunteers, the RNLI Heritage team and regional fundraising team all working together on a project to completely redevelop the museum.

Brenda was at the heart of the action. As a woman who shares with lifeboat crews a great quality of modesty, she would demur. Those who worked with her on the project remember otherwise. Firstly, she contributed to the planning of the new facility – known to be a person with definite and always very practical ideas, Brenda contributed enthusiastically at all the meetings. Brenda, though, is a great 'doer', and when practical help was needed she was always the first to volunteer. She is remembered by the RNLI Heritage team as the person who worked with them throughout a late November day in 2005 to pack up the collection: 'It was a bitterly cold day and the wind was blowing off the sea straight into the building because the door kept bursting open. Brenda never mentioned the cold, packed all day and cheerfully told stories to keep up our morale,' recall Joanna and Carolyn.

Brenda shared everyone's satisfaction and pride in the renovated Grace Darling Museum, and is delighted that it is attracting so many visitors to the area, benefiting the local community as well as the RNLI. After more than forty years of giving willingly, her enthusiasm remains as strong as ever.

Vera Robinson MBE

Now just a few years off her 100th birthday, Vera Robinson has given a lifetime of support to the RNLI. She joined the local Ladies' Lifeboat Guild when she was sixteen, as that was the minimum age at which she could help collect money on Flag Days. She is still a member of the guild and, across the eighty years of her membership, has taken the key roles of Treasurer, Secretary and Chairman. Now she is the Guild President.

Nowadays, the guild is mainly concerned with raising cash for the RNLI by means of Flag Days, coffee mornings and similar events, but in the past the ladies used to provide food, hot drinks and shelter for people who had been rescued until they could return to their homes. They also used to help repair and maintain protective clothing worn by the lifeboat crews. Vera can remember spending many hours knitting the long woollen sea boot socks worn by the crew.

Vera's contribution extends way beyond her fundraising achievements – she has taken a vital role in saving important lifeboat heritage. Known locally as a 'venerable historian', she has an exceptional knowledge of local history and has written twelve books and given innumerable presentations about Redcar. Living all her life in Redcar, she cares deeply about conserving the treasures of its past. On more than one occasion when the historic Redcar lifeboat, the *Zetland*, was under threat, Vera has taken a lead in the efforts to save it. Built in 1802 by Henry Greathead, the *Zetland* is the world's oldest lifeboat. It served at Redcar for almost seventy-eight years and saved 500 lives. Following its final service in 1880 the lifeboat was kept in Redcar, but organising appropriate display facilities was ever a

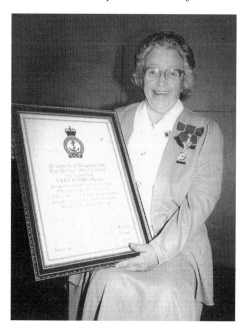

Vera Robinson proudly shows some of the awards she has received for her exceptional service to the RNLI.

recurring problem. This troubled people like Vera, who knew how significant the lifeboat was both for Redcar, and for lifeboat history in general.

In 1957, she provided the inspiration for members of the Ladies' Guild to re-open the boathouse in which the *Zetland* had been languishing uncared for during the war years. A lot of hard, physical work clearing and cleaning was done by the ladies. Amongst the dust and cobwebs they discovered a number of interesting artefacts which, after cleaning, were put on display. To manage the museum, it was decided to establish a separate Zetland Museum Committee. Not surprisingly, Vera was a leading light in the group, taking responsibility for the rota of volunteers who ran the whole operation.

This arrangement worked until 1969, when local government changes in the area led to a takeover of the museum by the local council. All worked well for a while, but the museum was closed in 1980. With her usual energy, Vera joined the local campaign to save the Zetland Museum. It was successful, and now the museum – once again run by volunteers – is a real asset for Redcar. Also for the RNLI, as it receives all the money from collecting boxes placed in the museum – a great source of satisfaction for Vera!

Many schools visit the Zetland Museum and Vera tells them the story about the boat, emphasising that the crew, like modern-day lifeboat crew, were not paid but were volunteers, ready to go out in all sorts of weather, day or night, to save anyone in distress at sea. She endeavours to tell them 'what an honour it is, to have in our keeping this wonderful boat'.

Vera has received a number of awards for the service she has given to her community and to the RNLI. The MBE was awarded in 1972 for working forty-two years as a teacher. Having already received Silver and Gold Badges from the RNLI, she received the organisation's highest volunteer award – Honorary Life Governor – in 1993. In 2001 she was conferred with the Freedom of the Borough of Redcar. These awards have brought Vera pride and pleasure, but they have never dimmed her enthusiasm to continue: 'Every time I get an award, I'm always asked: are you going to retire? But what would I do?' It is impossible to think that she will ever stop giving, either to her community, or to the RNLI.

Diana Alcaraz

Diana Alcaraz answers the question about why she has supported the RNLI for over forty years with a very poignant story. It relates to the outstanding service given by the RNLI to her husband – and to herself – in 1975.

Diana Alcaraz and her husband Paul, taken
shortly before he died.

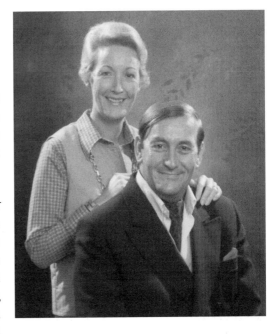

In that year Paul, who was a Spaniard
working in the city as a Re-insurance
Broker and with a passion for blue water
sailing, was diagnosed with lung cancer.
Diana relates:

> He tried to accept the constraints of
> his illness and sold his beloved boat. He
> managed for three weeks and then the
> brochures and sailing magazines came
> out and he announced that he had found
> a junk rigged sloop in Poole. The boat,
> named *Djong* (Burmese for Junk), had a
> self-steering vane, which meant he could
> operate the boat from the cockpit without having to manage heavy sails.
>
> He assured me that he had organised a crew to help him bring the boat back from Poole
> to Bembridge but I was uncertain from the outset and then when I realised he had made the
> decision to have one last voyage alone, I panicked.
>
> I rang Mike Attrill's boatyard at Bembridge and Mike rang the coastguard to explain. In turn
> the coastguard called the RNLI at Poole who promised to shadow Paul all the way home, pass-
> ing on responsibility to Yarmouth and then to Bembridge Lifeboats.
>
> Paul nearly made it. He got as far as Ryde Marina and collapsed. He couldn't go any further.
> Attrills brought the boat back to the yard with Paul onboard.

When Diana tells this story she sets great store not only by what the lifeboat crews did, but
how they did it, knowing that Paul was dying:

> No-one said that he was mad, no-one said what a blithering idiot he was. They understood
> what he was trying to do and how important it was for him to have one last voyage. No-one
> tried to force him to take on a crew, or to be towed into harbour. They cared and they under-
> stood.

Diana supports the RNLI not only because of her eternal gratitude for this understanding
and compassion for her husband, but also because such caring is at the very heart of crew
values:

> They care when no-one else cares. We need to know that someone else cares enough to
> put their lives on the line. They fill an enormous gap in our society with such integrity and
> sincerity.

After her husband died, Diana had a big responsibility to provide for her four children, but once they became independent she made provision in her will for a legacy for the RNLI. After attending an event for legacy pledgers at Headquarters, she realised how important it was to spread the word about legacy giving, and volunteered to be one of a group of volunteer speakers to represent the RNLI locally.

Diana enjoys this, and believes it to be a very fruitful way of giving support. She has a particular story that she always includes in her presentation. It relates to the days when she helped on RNLI collection days in Portsmouth:

> I was standing outside Tesco's on a Bank Holiday Friday doing a bucket collection in a fairly rough area. This little old lady, balancing two sticks, came up to me. 'In my pocket,' she said. 'I beg your pardon?' I said. 'In my pocket,' she repeated. I was aware that it would probably look as if I were mugging a fragile old lady, but I felt in her pocket and pulled out a five pound note. 'Put it in the bucket!' she said. 'Are you sure, that is a lot of money?' I said. She told me that she always gave this sum to the RNLI because 'They didn't manage to save him'.

The story that followed made me so glad that I had met her. Her father had been a fisherman and one night in a terrible storm he was washed overboard. The alarm was raised and the lifeboat was launched. They searched for six hours, but with no luck – he had disappeared. In spite of the dreadful weather, they carried on searching until fuel and exhaustion meant they had to return to harbour. She said they came to tell her mother how sorry they were they could not find him. Both she and her mother had been very worried that the crew were in danger that night, and so she always put money aside for her gifts to the RNLI.

Diana concludes her presentation by saying that a story like this – not of a big or dramatic rescue that hits the headlines and attracts huge publicity, but one the showing kindness, dedication and professionalism of these RNLI volunteer crews – proves that 'our people are heroes in the truest sense of the word'.

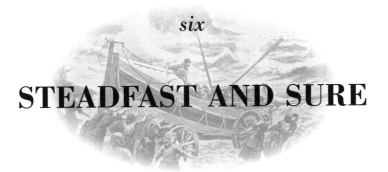

six

STEADFAST AND SURE

Women watching and waiting

It is hard to imagine that there is anyone who has not experienced the anxiety of waiting to know that a loved one has returned home safe. For some this may be hearing that visiting relatives have made the return journey home, or for parents that a teenager is back indoors after a night clubbing; for many families it is knowing that their son or daughter is safely home from deployment in a war zone. We have all tasted the flood of relief that comes when our worst fears have happily proved unfounded.

Who could conceive how it feels for women who know that their loved ones knowingly and willingly put their own lives at risk to go to the aid of others? What is it like to be waiting and wondering for hours on end if the lifeboat will return safely with all its crew intact? Moreover, what is it like to have this experience not once or twice in a lifetime, but regularly? Frequently, even? There are many women around our coast who do not need to imagine this situation; for them, such waiting is their reality. They are the wives, mothers, sisters, girlfriends, grandmothers, aunts and cousins of all those who crew our lifeboats.

From its first beginnings right up until today, the families of lifeboat crews have given steadfast support to their men – and more recently their women – for them to go to sea when the call came to launch the lifeboat. Often this would be in conditions so dangerous that most people would think it madness to go on to the beach, let alone set out to sea in a small boat. The courage of lifeboat crews is most surely matched by the courage of their loved ones, who understand what drives the need of some to help save lives at sea.

Home support for a crew member goes way beyond the experience of anxiety. For many, years having a husband and father on the crew, particularly if they were the coxswain, meant family life was significantly disrupted and real sacrifices had to be made by all. Many women describe their involvement more as a 'way of life' and find they become drawn into all sorts of activities such as fundraising and local promotion of the RNLI. Such closeness and sharing explains why many references are made with pride to the 'RNLI family'.

Solidarity within the RNLI family is poignantly shown when the worst happens – as tragically it has on a number of occasions. When an individual or a whole crew is lost on

A turn-of-the-twentieth-century lifeboatman bids farewell to his family. (Our Proud Heritage)

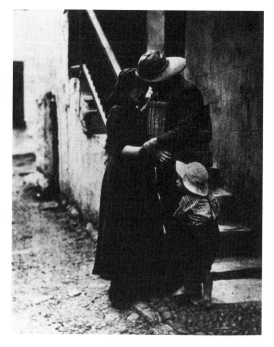

service, those who understand the best are both quickest to respond and longest to stay in support.

Wives and mothers

Nansie Evans – wife of Dick Evans BEM, former coxswain of Moelfre lifeboat

Dick Evans, a legendary RNLI coxswain and holder of two Gold Medals, was always very firm in his acknowledgment of how much the support of his wife had meant to him. Nansie was a farmer's daughter and claimed not to be particularly interested in the sea, but she knew Dick's life ambition was to be coxswain of the Moelfre lifeboat. Even though this meant long hours of separation – even going separately to chapel – she did not deter him. As coxswain's wife, she had to answer the telephone and take down instructions from the coastguard when a lifeboat launch was requested. Dick was proud that although some of the messages were complicated, his wife never once made a mistake.

Nansie lived with her fear when her husband and his crew went out to sea. She kept her thoughts to herself until hearing about the loss of the Longhope crew in 1969. Dick was deeply affected by this tragedy because he and the Longhope coxswain, Dan Kirkpatrick, were close friends. In these exceptional circumstances, Nansie disclosed her thoughts: 'Every time he put out I had that feeling that something was going to happen. For years it never did and they always came home safely. But that feeling was always there'.

Gloria Marsh – wife of Vic Marsh BEM, former coxswain of Swanage lifeboat

The Marsh family are well known in Swanage – they have been there for generations, operating boats for sightseeing and fishing trips. Gloria's husband Vic followed the family tradition in loving the sea, but for most of his working life he was employed by the RNLI first as the mechanic, then later becoming coxswain/mechanic of Swanage lifeboat. When he retired in 1990 he was awarded the BEM for his services in saving lives at sea.

Gloria, who met Vic when he was a young man, was not surprised when he told her of his intention to volunteer for the crew. His grandfather, Thomas Marsh, had been a lifeboat man, almost losing his life when, in 1895, he was washed overboard from the lifeboat. In this incident, the coxswain drowned – the only tragedy ever to have struck the lifeboat community of Swanage. Vic, who had trained as a plumber, joined the crew and was bowman.

He later took the opportunity to apply for the paid position of mechanic and was successful. Gloria was very supportive of her husband's passion for the lifeboat, and it was not long before she was involved. Her life was to be affected quite significantly.

It started with a request to help with the collection on Lifeboat Day, and not long afterwards Gloria joined the Ladies' Lifeboat Guild, becoming the Souvenir Secretary for a number of years. When the coastguard requested a lifeboat launch they made a telephone call to Vic and Gloria's home, and they had developed a good routine for a fast response. If it came at night, Vic immediately got dressed so that he could get to the boathouse as soon as possible to set off the maroons. Meanwhile Gloria was working her way through the crew list, telephoning them to say that a launch had been requested. This way, many of the crew were able to get there before they even heard the maroon. Gloria would then get dressed herself and make her way to the boathouse to put on the kettle in readiness to make hot drinks for the launchers and for the wet and weary crew when they returned. She remembers grabbing food from the house so that she could prepare something for them to eat. Sometimes, when she thought it would be a long rescue, she even took her own microwave in the car! She became renowned for her homemade bread pudding, which the coastguard enjoyed too.

A special request for even more of her help came when it was realised how distressing it was for some of the crew wives not to know what was happening to their husbands when the lifeboat launched. Gloria was asked by the Honorary Secretary to telephone each wife from the boathouse to tell them what was known about the incident and how long it might take and to keep them updated. She became the main point of information for the wives for about eighteen years – a huge commitment of her time.

Gloria recalls how she and the Swanage wives were certainly anxious for their husbands' safety, but says this was balanced by their total confidence in their men who they knew to be highly competent. At social events the wives would exchange thoughts, but they were always positive ones, full of support and enthusiasm for the crew's achievements. They felt an immense sympathy when lifeboat crew from other parts of the coast were lost, but could not help being relieved that it had not been their lifeboat.

When Gloria married Vic, she not only joined the large Marsh family, she also joined the extensive RNLI family – not just in Swanage, but all around our coastline. She first fully appreciated this when, after a long and tiring summer season, Vic encouraged her to take a holiday. She decided to visit some of the castles in Wales – castles are one of her passions. She was warmly welcomed when she put her head round a lifeboat house door in North Wales to say hello. In no time at all she was invited to meet Dick Evans, the famous retired coxswain of Moelfre lifeboat. Gloria well knew the name of this outstanding man and was amazed to think she might actually meet him. Both Dick and his wife, Nansie, greeted her as a long lost friend and were very hospitable, even though they were in the middle of having their house decorated. Undaunted, Dick found all his medals and vellums which had been carefully packed away and explained them all to Gloria. Invitations from other lifeboat stations followed, and so it was that Gloria's tour of castles became a tour of lifeboat stations.

Vic died in 1997, but he and Gloria passed on their passion for the lifeboat to their children and grandchildren. Their second son, Ian, joined the crew as soon he was old enough

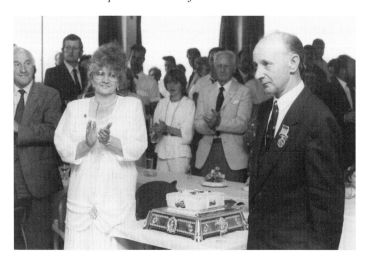

Gloria Marsh with her husband Coxswain Vic Marsh, Swanange, at the presentation of his BEM in 1990.

and very much hoped to follow his father into the mechanic/second coxswain role. Sadly this was thwarted when it was discovered that he was colour blind, and much to his distress, he was compelled to leave the crew. Eldest daughter Karina is married to the present coxswain, Martin Steeden. Their eldest son Gavin is on the crew and is a member of the RNLI Rapid Response Unit. In 2009 he went with them to assist the flood relief operation in Cumbria. Their second son, Matthew, is on the crew and is employed by the RNLI as a mechanical engineer, and James, son of second daughter, Belinda, is also on the crew. The tradition gets even stronger as great grandchildren start to appear, and where do the family choose to christen their babies? Swanage lifeboat, of course!

Gloria was awarded the RNLI Silver Badge for her service in 1987 and has continued with her support ever since, becoming President of the Ladies' Lifeboat Guild this year. She would not dream of doing otherwise. She joined with her husband in helping save the lives of others by giving practical support at the lifeboat station at all hours of the day and night. She is a woman who will speak sympathetically of the anxieties experienced by crew wives when their husbands are risking their lives, but is modest about her own worries and her husband's courage – a man awarded a Bronze Medal for his bravery. She says it has been an honour, and one she does not regret for one moment. With children and grandchildren following on from Vic, it seems that she has many more moments to come.

Julie Davies – wife of Richard Davies, former coxswain of Cromer lifeboat, and mother of John Davies, current coxswain of Cromer lifeboat

Richard Davies had always been passionate to join the lifeboat, and when he was just sixteen years old, became a member of the Cromer crew and subsequently their coxswain fourteen years later. He comes from a long line of Cromer lifeboat men, among them 'Shrimp' Davies who was a nephew of Henry Blogg, the RNLI's most decorated coxswain who served on the Cromer lifeboat for fifty-three years. Richard followed the strong Cromer tradition of being a volunteer coxswain and earned his living as a fisherman. For much of Julie's married life her husband has been on the sea in either a lifeboat or a fishing boat.

Julie says that it was essential to accept this as a way of life very early on in marriage, but that does not mean to say it was always easy. She would be continually watching the weather, dreading the sound of a gale or high seas knowing that her husband would be on the alert in expectation that his crew would get a shout. When they did respond to a call, her mind was always with him and she would say a little prayer. It was a fact that any personal or family plans could be changed by a single telephone call or by the maroons going off. Julie says that there were never any bad feelings about the lifeboat taking precedence: 'When you marry a fisherman and lifeboatman this should go without saying – that is their way of life, so you accept it. I have watched relations go wrong when this hasn't happened.'

Mobile phones help crews to keep in contact with their families today, but there were none when Richard was coxswain. Julie relied on tuning into the ship to shore radio and then she telephoned the other wives to share the news and give a likely time of return home. She can recall how she listened out for the men speaking – when she heard urgency in the tone, there was reason to be concerned. It was even worse if they temporarily lost communications, as once happened when she and Richard were listening to Wells-next-the-Sea lifeboat while it was on a tough service. She remembers that as a very frightening time. She could give practical help to the crew families by looking after their children and pets if the mother had to be at work while the men were on a rescue. It was all about supporting each other.

The anxious times that wives shared were balanced by the fun times they enjoyed together at many social events. Julie, with other wives, belonged to the Ladies' Guild, which was successful in raising lots of money. Often she would accompany her husband when he was called upon to receive a cheque for the RNLI. Understandably, people were always keen to meet the coxswain!

Now that Richard is retired, Julie still has anxiety when the lifeboat is out, for, just like his father before him, their son John could not wait to join the crew and did so as soon as he was seventeen. For a time both father and son were on the crew together – a big challenge for Julie's long held approach of accepting that this is the way things are: 'Having the two most precious men in my life both there together, I tried not to worry too much as I knew that was their wish' – but she did! She reflects that maybe it was because Richard was already on the crew and was a fisherman when she met him that it seemed easier to accept the danger he went into.

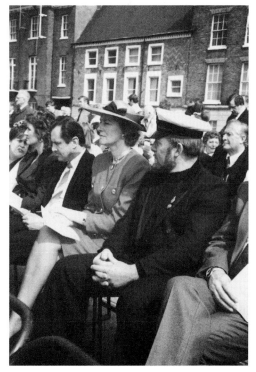

Julie Davies with her husband Richard Davies, former Coxswain of Cromer, attending a ceremony at Great Yarmouth Docks.

How proud she and Richard are that John was voted by the crew to follow in his father's footsteps as coxswain. Through all the worrying times and all the good times she has experienced in the last thirty-six years, Julie says that her pride in her husband, her son and all the RNLI crews has been constant.

Kathleen Davies – Cromer lifeboat in the Second World War

Throughout the war, Cromer lifeboat was kept very active in the busy sea-lanes of the east coast. With the threat of attack from bombs and mines, wives of the crew had even greater reason to be anxious when the lifeboat was launched.

Kathleen, wife of Henry Davies, has a poignant story about a lifeboat rescue that Henry Blogg and the Cromer crew undertook in October 1941. They went to the rescue of forty-four men on a ship aground on a sandbank twenty miles off the Cromer coast. Conditions were appalling – heavy seas and a bitterly cold wind. Having reached the casualty, Coxswain Blogg judged that it was too dangerous to try to put the lifeboat alongside the ship, so he decided to wait for a change in the tide. Two hours later he moved the lifeboat carefully towards the ship but was hit by a vast wave, with the outcome that five crewmen were flung into the cold water, one of whom was Henry Davies. All the men were pulled back onto the lifeboat and the coxswain took the lifeboat with the soaking men back to Cromer. Tragically one of them, 'Boy Primo' Allen, later died as a consequence of the time he spent in the icy water.

Waiting at home for news, Kathleen Davies became very anxious about the length of time the lifeboat was away. Suddenly she could bear it no longer, so took herself and her two young children to find the companionship of some other crew wives. She cared for her husband when he returned home sodden, cold and tired. Later, emptying his pockets in readiness to wash the clothes, she found his watch, which had stopped at 2.30 when he was swept overboard and exactly the time she had left home certain that the lifeboat was in trouble.

All forty-four men were subsequently rescued by the Cromer lifeboat.

Margaret Taylor – wife of Graham Taylor, former coxswain of Filey lifeboat

Some of Margaret's earliest memories are of lifeboats, and of sea and sand. When she was three years old her father, Richard Mason, took his family to live on Spurn Point so that he could join the crew of Humber lifeboat as second coxswain. His brother, John, was the coxswain. For their wives it was a hard life. They had no mains electricity; sand blew in through every door and window of the house; and their washing always dried stiff and hard because of the salt spray. If that wasn't enough, they had a constant battle with rabbits, who raided the vegetable patches and tried to get into the house. Once a week a bus took them on the sixteen-mile round trip to the shop. Self-sufficiency was absolutely essential. Fortunately, the children had more fun with great freedom to roam and play. When they left Spurn Head, none of them had any concept of the dangers of road traffic.

When the family eventually moved to Filey, Margaret's father took up fishing. One of the younger fishermen in the town, Graham Taylor, had been asked by Coxswain 'Dag' Chapman to join the crew and Margaret's father added his encouragement. Graham and

Margaret were later to marry, but during their courtship Margaret was to learn just how important the lifeboat had become for him. While on a romantic country walk, he heard the maroons go off and immediately rushed away to the boathouse. Margaret was left completely alone in the pitch dark and had to make her own way home. It was an early indication of how much her married life was to be dominated by the lifeboat service.

Soon after their wedding, the Ladies' Lifeboat Guild invited the new young crew wife to wash up at their fundraising events. Margaret looks back on this with great amusement; she was the first crew wife to be invited and she recalls that she actually felt honoured. She remembers a few years later the ladies' reaction to her offer to run a stall at the Christmas Fair – 'well you can try!' was the lukewarm answer. Undaunted, she did try, and did extremely well. In fact it was such a success that in no time she was running four stalls a year selling handmade items that she had knitted or sewn herself. Her beautiful work became so well known that customers placed orders to make sure they were not disappointed. Margaret's craft and needle skills have raised many thousands of pounds for the RNLI since her first stall in 1976.

Graham progressed on the crew to be second mechanic and was subsequently appointed as full-time station mechanic employed by the RNLI. In 1998 he became coxswain/mechanic, a position he held for ten years. Margaret recalls that while she was very proud of her husband, the job did have a big impact on their family life. Graham had few opportunities to go out for the day with his wife and children in case the lifeboat was needed. Margaret remembers occasions when, even though he had a properly approved day off, if Graham heard the maroons, he would turn back from the family and go to the boathouse. Margaret remembers one occasion very well:

> Graham was on leave and we were staying at home because we couldn't afford to go away. We were woken up very early by a fisherman asking Graham to use the lifeboat tractor for a coble which had become stuck in the sand. Feeling this to be unfair because Graham's deputy could do it, I rang my in-laws to ask if we could go to stay with them for a holiday and my father-in-law agreed to come and get us. While loading up the car, Graham heard the maroons go off and he vanished. Fortunately it was a false alarm, so Graham returned and we had our holiday.

Knowing a lot about the sea and the dangers faced by lifeboat crews, Margaret's natural instinct was to worry when her husband was out on a rescue, but when they married Graham had made her promise him that she would not worry. He explained that if he worried about her worrying about him, he could not concentrate while at sea. In return she made Graham promise that he would always wear his lifejacket. Margaret did her very best to honour her promise, but it was not always easy. One difficult time was when she was in the boathouse after the lifeboat was launched. As she looked out to sea, she could see the lifeboat vanishing in the troughs of huge waves. Then on the boathouse radio she heard the Station Honorary Secretary speaking to the lifeboat. His message was 'Filey lifeboat take extreme care'. They were chilling words for a wife to hear. Margaret says: 'I left the boathouse with my baby daughter and went home. It was a feeling I'll never forget.'

Margaret confirms being a lifeboat crew wife is a big commitment – one which requires women to be very understanding in spite of their inevitable frustrations. She has thrown

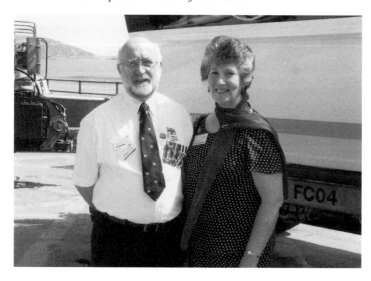

Margaret Taylor with her husband Graham Taylor, former coxswain of Filey, on the occasion of a visit by RNLI President the Duke of Kent, in 2006.

her heart and soul into supporting Filey lifeboat crew; she has brewed endless cups of tea on their return to the boathouse, whatever time of day or night, been a willing listener and been a mighty fundraiser. Graham is now retired, but both continue their support with undiminished energy and enthusiasm – he as a Deputy Launching Authority, and she as Vice Chairman of the Ladies' Guild. 'We'll never finish with the RNLI,' says Margaret.

Karen Steenvorden – wife of David Steenvorden, superintendent coxswain of Humber lifeboat

Humber Lifeboat Station is unique among the 235 stations operated by the RNLI because it is permanently manned by paid employees. The crew and their families must live at the end of a 3.5-mile road that runs the length of the sandy, shingle spit called Spurn Head. It is certainly a wild and isolated spot for human beings, but it is the perfect place to locate a lifeboat close to the deep water channel into the Humber Estuary. There has been a lifeboat here since 1802 and many generations of men, women and children have lived in the cottages since 1819.

Currently there is a full-time crew of seven men who, together with their families, add up to twenty-nine people living on Spurn Point. The limitations imposed by this extreme environment affect every aspect of domestic life; the nearest shop is eight miles away in Easington, as is the infant school. Older children have a longer journey to Withernsea, which is sixteen miles away. The single-track tarmac road is the fragile lifeline, but it can be breached by the sea, making it impassable on some occasions. This means that no one can go anywhere until the water recedes. This makes for a very distinctive lifestyle, and one which would not suit everyone! Sometimes the school bus cannot make it down the road so the children have to be taken in the RNLI Landrover up the 3.5 miles to meet the bus. The families can do nothing when the forces of nature take the road away from them – they just have to watch and wait. Another practical problem is living with the sand, which gets into everything. Washing machines do not last long on Spurn Point, Karen observes.

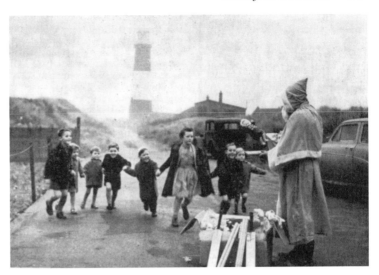

Father Christmas
arrives at Humber
Lifeboat Station in
1973. (*Yorkshire Post*)

Karen, wife of Superintendent Coxswain Dave Steenvoorden, has lived at Spurn Point for twenty years and has raised their two sons there. As a coxswain's wife she is more than familiar with the anxieties of 'watching and waiting', which she accepts philosophically as part and parcel of their life together. Like all the other crew wives who have ever lived at Spurn Point, she has had to make greater allowances than usually expected from a woman in support of her husband's work. 'You either love it or hate it,' says Karen. It is very clear that (for most of the time!) she loves it and has total commitment to the work of the crew in saving lives.

Designated as a nature reserve, Spurn Head is very peaceful. There is virtually no traffic and deer, foxes and rabbits all roam freely. Most visitors are those that appreciate natural things: birdwatchers; fishermen; walkers. Happily, it is still a relatively safe place for young children to play and they certainly enjoy a freedom that would be difficult elsewhere. Karen and Dave's sons thought it a paradise until they reached teenage years, and then they felt trapped. They wanted to join in with the activities their school friends were enjoying, but it was difficult. 'Whenever they wanted to go anywhere, I had to take them and they began to regard Spurn as a godforsaken place,' remembers Karen. 'I spent many hours as a taxi driver, to and from Scouts and other activities. The worst thing was waiting outside discos at 2.30a.m.' Now adults, they love the place again and are keen to come and visit their old haunts.

Living in such a small, isolated community could become like a goldfish bowl, but over the years Karen has learned some helpful lessons. The most important, she says, is to let the children sort out their own arguments – if adults get involved, the hurt can go deeper and be remembered long after the children are best of friends again. The seven families do enjoy social occasions together and the wives definitely enjoy a girls' night out, but it is important not to be socialising all day, every day. Helping a new family to make the necessary adjustments to such an unusual lifestyle is important too, and Karen makes sure they know that there is support. The best meeting place for them all is the small café, which Karen has been running for the past sixteen years. She mainly serves visitors to Spurn Point, but it is also the unofficial crew room – where the men come for breakfast after a shout, where the children drop in and out, and where their mothers can catch up with each other.

As a superintendent coxwain's wife, Karen usually learns first-hand about the launches and rescues, and she is able to communicate what she has learnt to the other wives. She well remembers how much she herself worried in the early days, and wants to do all she can to ensure the others have as much information as possible. Sometimes this is difficult, as it is typical of their husbands to say little. 'They keep a lot to themselves and will only tell their family what they need to know.' She believes that this is because lifeboat crew do not seek attention or praise for themselves. In fact, 'they are a breed of their own' she says.

The safety of their husbands is always at the front of their minds. None of them can ever become blasé about that. Always, though, they share the rejoicing in the lives saved by their lifeboat crew. As Humber Lifeboat Station reaches its 200th anniversary in 2010, 1,550 people have been saved.

Daughters

Vera Cross MBE – daughter of Robert Cross, former coxswain of Humber lifeboat

Memories of life on Spurn Point are still very clear for Vera Cross, who in 1918 was born daughter to Coxswain Robert Cross and his wife, Sarah. She recalls how cold and draughty it was in the old cottage, which had no electricity. Sand blew in through the many cracks in the building and got everywhere – even in their food. Even now, Vera remembers the gritty texture in her mouth. She was an only child – a very precious one, her parents told her, but had the company of about thirteen other children whose fathers served with Robert Cross on the lifeboat crew. They all played freely on the beach and among the dunes – there was no reason for their parents to worry about them. One thing was forbidden though; they were never allowed to go on the lifeboat! Vera confirms that it must have been a very

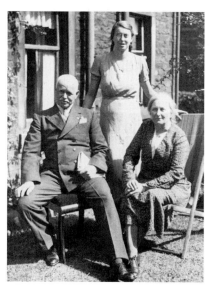

hard life for the families living on Spurn in those days, but she is adamant that they were all accepting of what seemed quite natural to them. That their fathers and husbands were saving lives was all-important, and a source of great pride.

The only telephone was in the coxswain's house. It was installed in her parents' bedroom, and to it came the calls requesting a lifeboat launch. Vera relished the special task her father gave her when he asked her to lay out the nautical charts he needed

Vera Cross with her father, Coxswain Robert Cross, Humber, and her mother, Sarah, in Bradford in 1954 when Coxswain Cross was invited to the city to receive the lifeboat *City of Bradford III*, which had been funded by the people of Bradford.

to plot his course to a casualty. She felt that she was helping this brave man who so inspired her. In those days, the families received no communication from the lifeboat while it was on a rescue and they never knew when it would return. They were anxious hours for many, but Vera recalls never being afraid because she had such faith that they would return. She knew her father to be highly respected by his crew, even though all were men of few words.

Robert Cross received seven RNLI medals and additionally the George Medal in 1940. He was without question one of the RNLI's most outstanding coxswains, operating in dangerous waters and performing daring rescues throughout the Second World War. During his time of service on the Humber lifeboat, 453 lives were saved. When he retired in 1943, he and his wife went to live in Withernsea and were joined by Vera who had secured employment as secretary at the local school. She cared for both her parents until they died and worked at the school until her own retirement. She was awarded the MBE for her services to education.

Now living in a nursing home, Vera says her love and pride in her father has never diminished. On the wall next to her bed is a picture of him, looking very handsome in his coxswain's uniform and wearing all his medals. She looks at it frequently and still draws inspiration from him – every day.

Granddaughters

Amy Kneen – granddaughter of Edward Kneen, former coxswain of Port St Mary lifeboat

Amy is not a person to boast about her own achievements in supporting the RNLI all her life. She states quite simply that she had very good reason to do so. This is a reference to her father, William, and grandfather, Edward, who both served as crew on the Port St Mary lifeboat. Her poignant memory of how her grandfather tragically lost his life while in service has been a major motivator.

Amy, born in 1920, was his eldest and much loved grandchild. He enjoyed taking her with him when he did his weekly inspections of the lifeboat every Saturday. Amy's earliest memories are of being lifted into the lifeboat to find the sweets he had hidden there for her to find. She then watched him going about his routine checks.

'Teddy' Kneen lost his life on Port St Mary Lifeboat Day on 6 August 1927. Traditionally, the event was started by the release of a maroon, which would normally be the responsibility of the signalman on the crew to fire. On this occasion, knowing how short money was for him, Teddy had generously given him permission to work that day unloading a coal ship, saying he would fire the maroon himself. As he lit the fuse, there was a huge explosion. The shell flew straight at him, causing terrible injuries to his face and head. It was clear to all that there was absolutely no hope of recovery, so a message was sent to Teddy's wife telling her what had happened. Meanwhile he was lifted onto a handcart and taken to his home where his wife, also named Amy, was now anxiously awaiting her husband. The family sat with him until he died later that day.

Amy recalls that her family lost none of their commitment to the lifeboat service after this – if anything, it grew stronger. Her father continued to serve on the crew for a further

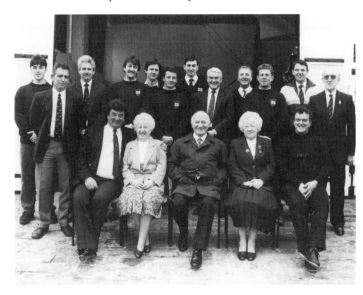

Amy Kneen (right)
with her sister Ann and
the crew and Station
Committee of Port St
Mary lifeboat in 1993.

thirty-three years. She and her sister, Ann, became strong supporters of the Port St Mary Ladies' Lifeboat Guild. When Amy retired as headmistress of a school in Staffordshire, she returned to the family home and first became Secretary and later Chairman and President of the Guild. As a little girl, her family had referred to her as 'The Organiser' – a skill Amy has used with great vigour to help raise many thousands of pounds for the RNLI.

'Adopted mothers'

Georgina Keen, St Peter Port Lifeboat Station

The boathouse at St Peter Port Lifeboat Station, Guernsey has the most unusual exhibition on its walls. A series of pictures of an elegant lady with a giant turkey – or turkeys – surrounded by lifeboat crew, all with smiles in anticipation of the feast ahead. What makes each picture so distinctive is that the huge wishbone is mounted in the frame, making a complete record of the happy occasion.

The elegant lady is Georgina Keen, who every year cooked a Christmas lunch for everyone involved with this lifeboat station. A tremendous undertaking for one person, but she relished this as one of the ways she could express her admiration and support for the work of the station. Peter Bisson, former coxswain of St Peter Port lifeboat, remembers that it all started with a drinks party thrown by Georgina for the crew in 1975. The party was enjoyed by all, but when Georgina learned that afterwards the boys went out for a meal she decided that she would make the event a dinner the following year. He is keen to correct the impression that Georgina cooked for them just once a year: 'Whenever we had a long shout, she would come down to the boathouse with bacon sandwiches. She cared for the crew and nothing was too much trouble for her when she was helping the boys.'

What is quite extraordinary about this is that Georgina held a very senior volunteer role in the RNLI. She was one of the first women to be appointed, in 1975, as a Vice President of the Committee of Management. She was a member of the fundraising committee from 1971–1992, and the establishment committee from 1979–1988. Clearly these positions brought significant responsibilities, but Georgina was not one to stand on her dignity – she made sure she was there with her 'hands on' practical support for men who were cold and hungry when they returned from sea.

Criccieth was where it all started. It was where Georgina's grandmother, had a house on the seafront and summer holidays were enjoyed there. The house was the perfect spot to see the lifeboat returning after a shout, and Elizabeth Wiley regularly took hot drinks for the crew to help them recover from the wet and cold conditions. Little Georgina helped and noticed how, in a small community, everyone cared about the crew and got involved to help in any way they could.

Living inland, the best way she could help was to get involved with local RNLI fundraising and so she joined Kidderminster Ladies' Lifeboat Guild and threw herself into everything with great gusto. She was enthusiastically supported by her husband, Arthur, who had a busy career but who liked to help Georgina by coming up with new ideas. Between 1971 and 1979, she produced five cookbooks, pulling together recipes sent to her from all over the country. They were popular sellers and made a good profit for the RNLI. She was awarded the RNLI Silver Medal in 1974.

Retirement to Guernsey in 1975 brought them both close to the sea and gave them the opportunity to become a real part of the lifeboat community. She joined the Guernsey Ladies' Lifeboat Guild, bringing her redoubtable energy and enthusiasm to everything she did. After an approach from the Guernsey Tomato Marketing Board, the next two cookery books, 'The Love Apple' and '101 Tomato Recipes', were all tomato based.

Georgina died unexpectedly in June 1996, only sixty-three years of age. Members of the St Peter Port lifeboat crew carried her coffin and the wider lifeboat community joined with her family and friends to give thanks for a very talented and big-hearted woman. She holds a significant place in their hearts for all the many acts of kindness she showed them while also having a key position in the national history of the RNLI as a pioneering senior volunteer.

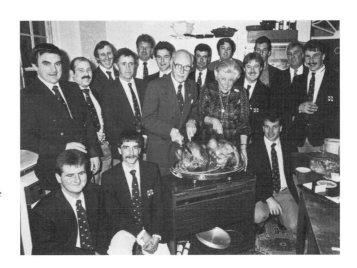

Georgina Keen with her husband, Arthur, ready to carve the massive turkeys she has cooked for the 1991 Guernsey Lifeboat Station Christmas lunch. (Brian J. Green)

Jo Allam BEM, Weston-super-Mare Lifeboat Station

In Weston-super-Mare she was known as 'The Lifeboat Lady', while at the lifeboat station Jo Allam was better known either as 'Mrs A' or to the crew as 'Mother'. These alternative names reflect the tremendous affection everyone felt for the woman who adopted the station and gave it her all for over fifty-three years.

It all started with the tragic loss of her husband, Patrick, who drowned when he was just twenty-six. He was the Chief Steward and Purser of the *Santampa*, which sank off the Welsh coast in the Bristol Channel on 23 April 1947. All forty-nine crew lost their lives. The tragedy was compounded by the loss of all eight men of the Mumbles lifeboat which launched to go to the rescue of the *Santampa*. Jo, widowed at such an early age with two small children to bring up, was deeply moved by the bravery and sacrifice of the Mumbles lifeboat crew, and decided that she would dedicate her life to the RNLI.

At Weston-super-Mare she took over responsibility for selling RNLI souvenirs at the lifeboat station and helping in any other way possible. She was a member of the Station Branch Committee, the Fundraising Committee and took on the role of Lifeboat Liaison Officer. It is hardly surprising that she became known locally as the 'Lifeboat Lady' – she involved herself in everything possible.

Jo did much more than just raise money at the shop and at events – she always had time for a cheerful conversation with her customers, explained the work of the crews and took those who were interested to see the old lifeboat station. She was a perfect ambassador for the cause, and who knows how many people gave generously to the charity thanks to her enthusiasm and commitment? The RNLI knew it had a very special supporter and thanked her with Silver and Gold Badges, and then with the ultimate accolade of Honorary Life

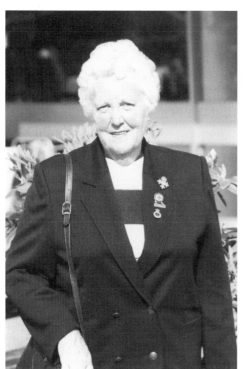

Governor in 1992. She was awarded the BEM in 1983.

Her devotion to the lifeboat crews is what earned her the name 'Mother'. There was nothing she would not do for them – immediately she knew the lifeboat had been launched, she arrived at the station, put the kettle on, made sandwiches and waited for the men to return so that she could take care of them. It was fortunate that she lived overlooking the station, but this may not have been a coincidence.

Her dedication to the crew meant that if any of them ever had a problem, it was to Jo they turned. She was kind, sympathetic and – very importantly – she could be completely trusted. Pete Holder, Lifeboat Operations Manager at Weston-super-

Jo Allam – the 'mother' of the Weston-super-Mare lifeboat crew – in 1995.

Mare, is but one member of her extensive fan club: 'Her door was always open, she was there for all of us, all of the time.' Nothing was too good for her boys, as RNLI HQ became well aware – a telephone call from Jo Allam to the Operations department meant prompt action would be needed to satisfy their intensely well meaning but outspoken 'Mother'!

In 2003 Jo decided to take a 'back seat' after fifty-three years, but she did not retire. She died in July 2007, aged eighty-five years. Saying farewell to this special person was a sad occasion for all at Weston-super-Mare Lifeboat Station. No one else had ever done so much for them. Her coffin was draped with the RNLI flag and carried by members of past and present lifeboat crew, and the chapel was packed with the many people who held Jo in the highest esteem. The decision about how and where to scatter her ashes was an easy one – at sea from the lifeboat, just off Birnbeck Lifeboat Station. The final words were 'Jo Allam, Mother to her RNLI Boys, Rest in Peace'.

Mary Taylor, Padstow Lifeboat Station

Mary comes from lifeboat stock and has calculated that her family has given 290 years of service to the RNLI. Her grandfather and father were both coxswains of Padstow lifeboat; two of her uncles also served on the crew, and her son, Eric, and grandson, James, have served on the crew at Penlee. Mary cherishes the Silver and Bronze Medals for gallantry awarded to her relatives. Her own contribution accounts for seventy-five years, and Mary's first memory of lifeboat service was when she was five years old, helping her mother with the lifeboat day collection: 'I was walking with the box through Padstow and saw some people coming towards me. All excited, I went up to them and said, 'Would you like to have a flag? My Daddy is the Coxswain'. 'Did they buy a flag?' I asked, and the answer came straight back: 'Of course they did!' In fact, people have been giving money to Mary for the lifeboat ever since, and she will be asking for as long as she has the breath to do so.

Mary has been resourceful in finding ways to extract money from people's pockets. She has organised bazaars and stalls, filling them with her handmade crafts, toys and embroideries, as well as a huge range of cakes, puddings and pastries. For many years, tourists to Padstow found her a familiar sight on the quay selling RNLI lottery tickets throughout the summer season. Perhaps her finest effort was when she sold raffle tickets for a linen tablecloth and matching napkins. She had embroidered these quite exquisitely with the RNLI insignia and the signatures of each of the lifeboat crew. 'I sold £12,000 worth of tickets and then I was told I would have to stop – I had reached my legal limit. Mind you, I could have got more.' This is a woman who does not give up easily. The money was used to help finance the new lift at the lifeboat station.

Mary explains that the story has an unexpected ending. The winning ticket was bought by a lifeboat enthusiast who was very happy with his fine prize. When he died several years later, his niece found the linen set in pristine condition and sent it back to Padstow Lifeboat Station. It is now used on very special occasions. Mary has a plethora of stories about her fundraising activities and tells them with enthusiasm: 'Once a photographer saw me going out with my boxes and said cheerfully, "I'll give you another 10 per cent of what you collect today".' This was a serious challenge for Mary who worked at the collecting all day and was thrilled to count £340 worth of coins at the end. 'The photographer pulled a face – it was much more than he expected. But he paid up!'

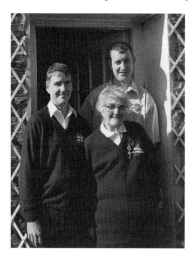

Mary Taylor – 'Lifeboat Mary' – of Padstow with her son Eric and grandson James.

To describe Mary as a fundraiser is to account for just a part of what she has committed herself to for the past seventy-five years. Much of her energy has been directed towards 'Looking after my boys'. By this she means going to the boathouse whenever there is a shout, day or night, and making sure there is food and drink for them on their return. In the early days this meant going home and carrying the pots of tea and food back. Now this can be done much more easily in the crew room. Her specialities are fried breakfasts, sandwiches and pickled onions! Coxswain Alan Tarby is quick to acknowledge how welcome this has been when returning cold, wet and tired. Mary says, 'It's nothing – it's just what I want to do for the boys. As long as I have them safe in the boathouse, I haven't got a care in the world'.

Mary has a ready knowledge of the history of Padstow Lifeboat Station. She says proudly that she has walked the decks of eleven of its eighteen lifeboats and, pointing to a picture on her wall of the lifeboat *Princess Mary* (stationed at Padstow 25 May 1929 to 25 July 1952), recounts how, as a girl, she used to swim out to the lifeboat, run around the deck and then dive from her back into the sea. Would she have joined the crew if it had been permitted in her day? 'Like a shot!'

No one could fail to recognise Mary's conviction about her way of doing things and it has not always made for an easy relationship with other local fundraisers. 'I know I am a one woman band,' she says. This one woman band has, however, raised tens of thousands of pounds, and the RNLI has recognised her service with awards of Gold and Bar to Gold Badges. In May 2010 she was presented with the highest volunteer award in the RNLI – Honorary Life Governor. Mary wonders if it will be presented by the Duke of Kent: 'Last time he presented me with a badge I asked him if he would like one of my cross stitch pictures of our lifeboat. He said he did not have enough wall space.'

In Padstow's boathouse there are eighteen beautiful counted cross-stitch pictures, one of each lifeboat to have served at the station. Such fine needlework represents hours and hours of this woman's time – and an immeasurable quantity of love for her coxswain and crew. It is no wonder that they affectionately call her 'Lifeboat Mary'.

Guernsey Women's Royal Voluntary Service (WRVS)

No one is quite sure who first had the idea, but it was such a good one that it gained enthusiastic support from all the members of the WRVS on Guernsey. What lay behind the idea of the WRVS giving support to the lifeboat crew? All its members are volunteers, and so there was an obvious resonance with the volunteers of the lifeboat crew. Both are charities and both are intensely practical in their approaches – it was a perfect match!

In 1952 Guernsey WRVS resolved that it would provide a cup of tea and a welcome whenever the lifeboat returned from a service call or exercise. They honoured this pledge for twenty years – a total of 150 tea-brewing occasions! Remarkably, a diary was kept of every occasion. Entries included the date, times, a brief description of the purpose of the launch, with details of what the lifeboat and its crew achieved. Also included were details of some of the practical challenges associated with receiving and responding to calls at all hours of the day and night, in all weathers and then to make and transport the tea to the boathouse to arrive in time for the return of the crew.

Some extracts from the diaries poignantly tell of the efforts made by this group of women to bring comfort and support to men arriving back at St Peter Port Lifeboat Station. They would often be tired, cold and wet, and in desperate need of a hot drink:

Saturday 26 December 1953: Service Call no. 7
… At 9.30p.m. call was received that one fishing boat had been found. At 10.15p.m. second call received, after which the team proceeded to the hut. Tea was served to one survivor, two members of the committee (RNLI) and crew; approximately twenty cups in all. Being Boxing Day Christmas cake and cigarettes were served. Team returned to HQ 11p.m.

Friday 2 July 1954: Service Call no. 10
… News was received at 11.30p.m. that a yacht was in distress … we then proceeded to HQ, got all in readiness, making tea at 1a.m. … we are pleased to report distressed craft was brought in safely and we proceeded to the lifeboat hut … forty-eight cups of very hot tea served. The welcome given us by the crew, States Supervisor, police and press was very gratifying. Remarks from the crew: 'have you a cigarette, we got through ours by 2a.m.' A box of fifty was handed round. We left White Rock at 5a.m., proceeded to HQ where all was left in readiness for next call. Left at 5.35a.m. – tired but very happy.

17 January 1957: Service Call no. 25
… Received call to say that lifeboat would be in harbour in half an hour. With that informa-tion we found that we had twenty minutes to make preparations which normally take half an hour … the water did not seem to boil fast enough and with every minute precious, Mrs

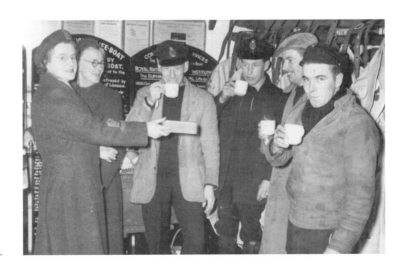

Guernsey WRVS attended every lifeboat shout from 1952 to 1972 and brewed tea for the crew on their return.

Ealand and I had visions that the lifeboat would be safely moored and the crew safely tucked in their beds before we would be able to put in an appearance. Oh, how dreadful. Our worries increased with that awful dread. Well, there was nothing we could do about it, and were able to leave HQ at 10.10p.m. arriving at the Hut at 10.15, very much relieved to find we were first and with time to spare … it was precisely at 10.45p.m. that the crew entered and although they are always delighted to see the WRVS, they were especially so on this occasion and each one spontaneously remarked, 'how nice we did not expect to see you because of petrol rationing'. Eighteen cups of tea were served.

17 February 1958: Service Call no. 30

At 6.30a.m. received call from Mrs Blampied that lifeboat was searching for a French trawler … 7.40a.m. second call and proceeded to HQ. Arrived at Hut at 8.15a.m. … served twelve cups of tea.

Hundreds of cups later, WRVS Guernsey performed their very last tea service on 29 August 1972 – a very special service and a very real contribution to helping the RNLI to save lives at sea.

Watching and waiting until your loved ones return home safely – or not at all

The truth behind the often quoted words 'lifeboat crews risk their lives to go to the rescue of others' has been proven many times. Every shout has the potential for something to go wrong – the sea is so unpredictable. Every crew household finds its own way of getting

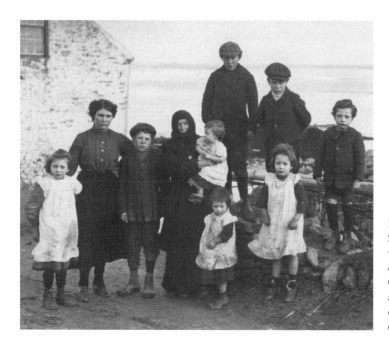

Fethard Lifeboat Station, 1914. The widow and nine children of Patrick Cullen, who drowned along with the whole crew of nine men during a rescue.

A page from *The Lifeboat Memorial Service Book.*

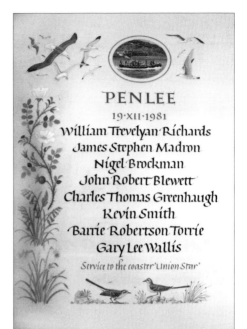

PENLEE

19·XII·1981

William Trevelyan Richards
James Stephen Madron
Nigel Brockman
John Robert Blewett
Charles Thomas Greenhaugh
Kevin Smith
Barrie Robertson Torrie
Gary Lee Wallis

Service to the coaster 'Union Star'

through what may be many hours while waiting for news of the safe return of the lifeboat and its crew. Fervent hopes that this shout will end well fades only when word comes that there has been a tragedy and life has been lost.

With his first-hand experience of the harsh realities of sea rescue, Sir William Hillary knew it was inevitable that men on lifeboats would lose their lives. His proposition included provision for widows and families to receive financial support, an essential support which has always been honoured. The Lifeboat Benevolent Fund provides pensions for widows and dependents equivalent to those paid when a chief petty officer in the Royal Navy is killed on active service.

The loss of precious lives while on lifeboat service has always been keenly felt by the wider RNLI family. A great desire to show solidarity with those bereaved is met by raising money to give them practical help. Many also feel a strong wish to commemorate those who have paid such a great price for the cause of saving life at sea. In most lifeboat communities where lives have been lost, there is a local memorial.

In the 1970s, Lord Saltoun, Convenor of the Scottish Council of Lifeboats, decided that there was a need for some form of national recognition. He raised the money to pay for *The Lifeboat Service Memorial Book* – a beautiful hand-illuminated record of every crew member who had lost his life on service since 1824. Composed of vellum sheets and bound by oak boards cut from the oak knees traditionally used for the stems of lifeboats, the book was created by The Society of Scribes and Illuminators. Containing 438 names, it is unquestionably a national treasure, but one which has to be looked after with great care, and which, unfortunately, is not on display to the public.

In 2006, Andrew Freemantle, then RNLI Chief Executive, took the lead in raising the funds and commissioning a memorial – a sculpture – naming everyone in the British Isles who had lost their lives in the cause of saving lives at sea. A total of 778 names are recorded on the memorial, which is situated adjacent to RNLI Headquarters in Poole.

Penlee lifeboat disaster

Understandably, the pain of a lifeboat disaster is felt for very many years within its community. Within the wider population, memories are not held for so long – probably with the exception of Penlee. Occurring just six days before Christmas in 1981, the disaster evoked great sympathy for the eight families in the tiny community of Mousehole in Cornwall. Each was coping with an unthinkable loss of a loved one at possibly the most difficult time of the year.

Led by Coxswain Trevelyan Richards, the Penlee lifeboat, *Soloman Browne*, was launched to go to the rescue of a ship, *Union Star*. It was drifting dangerously towards rocks after its engines had failed. It was reported that there were eight people on board. Conditions could not have been worse – the wind was blowing to hurricane force twelve and gusting to ninety knots, the sea was mountainous with waves reaching sixty feet high, and there was driving rain and poor visibility. All the experience and skill of Coxswain Richards and the crew was needed as they tried again and again to take the lifeboat alongside the *Union Star*. But the lifeboat was dwarfed by the huge waves, which slammed it hard against the side of the ship, even lifting the lifeboat up onto the deck only for it to slide stern first back into the sea.

Over an hour after the launch, a radio message was sent from the lifeboat confirming that four people had jumped from the ship into the lifeboat. The radio message was cut short as it was seen that the lifeboat turned back towards the ship, possibly to make another approach. No further communication came, but the lights of the *Soloman Browne* disappeared some ten minutes later. There were no survivors from either the ship or the lifeboat, and the timber-built lifeboat was smashed to small pieces.

The eight men of Penlee lifeboat crew who died that night were: Coxswain Trevelyan Richards; Second Coxswain/Mechanic James Stephen Madron; Assistant Mechanic Nigel Brockman; Emergency Mechanic John Robert Bluett; and crew members Charles Thomas Greenhaugh, Kevin Smith, Barry Robertson Torrie, and Gary Lee Wallis. The RNLI Gold Medal for outstanding gallantry was awarded to Trevelyan Richards and the Bronze Medal for gallantry to each member of the crew.

RNLI lifeboat crew are known for their courage, their modesty and dignity – as are their families. Theirs is a private grief, lived privately with a steadfastness and surety which is one of the clear hallmarks of RNLI families. It is a grief which, sadly – but predictably – some journalists have tried to exploit. Respect for their feelings and genuine concern to honour their wishes deters me from writing at length about the experiences of our widows and their families. Yet, theirs being so great a contribution to the cause of saving life at sea, I felt compelled to make a request to gain a better understanding of this profound experience. It was generously answered by Janet Madron, who lost her husband Stephen on the Penlee lifeboat nearly thirty years ago.

Janet Madron – wife of Stephen Madron, second coxswain/mechanic, Penlee lifeboat

Janet recalls that 19 December 1981 was, from the beginning, a very strange day. It started when Stephen got up, looked out of the window and called to her to come and see the beautiful sunrise. Feeling sleepy, she said no. 'Will you please come and look at this sunrise?' he repeated, but Janet stayed in bed. That afternoon Janet and Stephen, together with their four-year-old daughter Caron and son Ian, aged two, put up their Christmas tree. Actually they put up two, because the children wanted it that way. Stephen had bought some new decorations for the tree, including a peacock, which Janet still puts on her Christmas tree every year. When finished, Janet took Caron to a Christmas party but before she left, Stephen asked her to come back quickly, as he had heard there was a ship in trouble and the lifeboat might be needed.

Stephen Madron, second coxswain mechanic of
Penlee lifeboat.

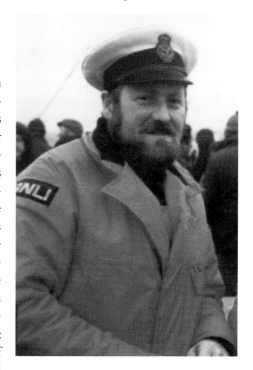

She did hurry back, and sure enough, soon
afterwards Stephen was called to the boathouse. Janet knew how bad the weather was
and for the first time ever was afraid for her
husband's safety. She said to him, 'Don't go –
I don't want you to go'. Stephen's reply was
simple: 'Got to go – there's women and children out there.' Then he was gone. From the
window of their house, Janet saw the lights
of the lifeboat dipping up and down in the
waves and then disappear from view. She
could not bear to look any longer so drew the
curtains. Stephen had left without eating his
dinner. Again, Janet remembers how strange
she felt as she put it in the oven to keep warm:
'I slammed it in the oven, saying to myself
"he's not coming back – he won't eat this". I'd
never done that before.'

Before long, two of their friends, Roy and Margaret Pascoe, arrived at the house. Roy
was a member of the lifeboat crew but had not been picked that night, so they came to sit
with Janet – something they had never done before when the lifeboat was out. Together
they listened on the scanner, which relays the radio communications with the lifeboat
while it is at sea. Janet heard Stephen's voice make the last transmission before the radio
went dead. From that moment she sensed the worst had happened. She listened to the
coastguard repeatedly calling the lifeboat, but there was no response.

Her memories of the rest of that night are far from complete. Janet remembers how desperately she wanted her dad and so a message was sent asking him to come. He had to walk
the two miles from Newlyn to Mousehole on a wild night, so it took some time for him to
arrive. When he did, he confirmed that he had walked along the top of the cliff looking for
the lifeboat but could see nothing. He went out again to search, but returned saying: 'No
man could live out there this night.'

They sat up all night waiting for news and were so tired and distraught the following day
that it was difficult to cope with the almost constant flow of people who came to express
their condolences. For days and weeks, people came to the house: family, friends, neighbours,
but also representatives from communities farther away. People meant so well, but it was all
very draining. Apart from this, Janet had difficult and painful things to do – breaking the
news to Stephen's parents was hard, particularly to his mother who loved him dearly. The two
young children had their world turned upside-down and desperately needed her attention.

There was huge media interest and some journalists were unscrupulous in how they
tried to obtain material from the bereaved families. One female reporter tried to force
her way into Janet's house but fortunately her sister-in-law was alert and managed to slam

the door shut in time. Looking back, Janet is clear that the love and support of her family saw her through the worst of her great loss. She refers to her father as 'My Rock' and her mother and brother did all they could, too. Janet has an identical twin sister, Jeanne, who came to live with her immediately and was a constant support. Janet's young nephew Nigel, who was only seven at the time, took hold of her hand one day and said: 'Don't worry Aunty Jan, I'll look after you.'

Help from the RNLI was important, too, and Janet remembers how kind and concerned the staff were to her. When Winston Graham, RNLI Director, visited her at home, she thought how proud Stephen would have been to see him there. Stephen had always been passionate about the RNLI. His grandfather had been coxswain at Penlee and his father had been on the crew. As a youngster he had volunteered as a 'runner' hoping to get on the crew if an extra hand were needed. On one of their early dates, Janet thought she had been 'stood up' when Stephen did not arrive at the agreed time. In fact, he was on a thirty-six-hour lifeboat service, going out to the grounded oil tanker, *Torrey Canyon*. The call came after he had dressed for their date, so he spent the whole time on the lifeboat in his best suit! After they were married, Janet was happy to support him when he got the opportunity to work full-time for the RNLI, even though the pay was low and they had to move house. She understood that lifeboating was in his blood.

Losing the love of your life in such tragic circumstances after only eleven years of marriage, and with the daunting prospect of raising two young children alone, is so devastating that most people would have understood if Janet had decided she wanted nothing more to do with the lifeboat service. But Janet remembers precisely when she made her decision

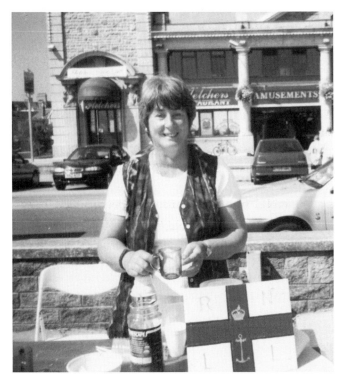

Janet Madron – busy fundraising for the RNLI.

about what to do. A few days after Stephen died, she suddenly felt a great need to see Mary Richards, mother of Coxswain Trevelyan Richards. Janet and Mary had been good friends for years; both enjoyed working on the Ladies' Guild and sharing each other's company when washing up together at fundraising events.

Mary, who was in her eighties when Trevelyan died, was staying at her daughter's house. For her, the loss of her son – such an able and well respected coxswain – was devastating. Janet's father accompanied her to the house and once the tea was made, they were thoughtfully left alone to talk. Straight away Mary said: 'Janet, what are we going to do about this lot?' She paused and then answered her own question; 'Well, I think we should carry on'. Janet recalls looking at the elderly lady and thinking, 'If Mary, as the coxswain's mother says this, then I can'.

Janet is quite clear that Mary Richards was her inspiration to carry on supporting the RNLI – which she has done with great energy ever since. As the Chairman of a very successful Ladies' Guild she oversees a busy fundraising calendar which includes a summer fête, a sponsored walk, teas for open gardens, a Flag Day, and helping in the lifeboat shop in Penzance. Last year the guild raised over £35,000 for the RNLI. Additionally, she gives talks to groups – both children and adults. She hopes that she is planting the seeds of future support wherever she goes.

Janet was awarded the Gold Badge in 2006, and after the celebrations with the crew and Ladies' Guild, went on her own to the peaceful garden that has been created around the old Penlee boathouse from which the *Soloman Browne* launched. There she looked out to sea and told Stephen and the crew that she had been given the Gold Badge. Going there over the years has helped Janet greatly.

The last thing she wants is to bring attention to herself. Her motivation is twofold; firstly, to honour the memory of Stephen in everything she does for the RNLI, and secondly, to help make enough money to ensure that today's crew always get the best of everything. It is this concern for them and the service they provide today that is so striking in Janet's approach to life. She likes the relationship she has at the boathouse, which means a warm welcome whenever she pops in. Her own children, Caron and Ian, give her their firm support and are as pleased as she is with all the opportunities that have come her way through the RNLI. Janet takes every chance to do interesting things like a practice helicopter winch and she loves meeting the many special people associated with the lifeboat service.

If it is at all possible to turn a negative into a positive, then Janet Madron of Penlee Lifeboat Station has definitely found the formula.

If you want to meet people in the RNLI who have immense courage, dedication and selflessness you will find these qualities in abundance – on the lifeboats and in the boathouses around our coastline. Look again more deeply, and you will find yet more within thousands of extraordinary women – those who stand steadfast and sure behind every crew volunteer.

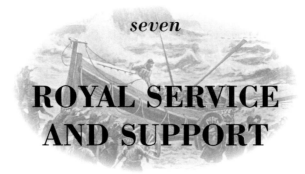

seven

ROYAL SERVICE
AND SUPPORT

Some may have thought him an idealist, but the great optimism of Sir William Hillary that a national lifeboat service would be supported from 'the palace to the cottage' was well founded. From 'the palace' has always come a ready understanding of the need for lifeboats and their crews around our coastline, and this has been underpinned with solid support for all RNLI volunteers. The female members of the royal family have been particularly generous in giving their time for formal events such as lifeboat naming ceremonies and medal presentations. The major contribution, though, derives from the special understanding of the volunteer ethos of the service that many of the royal women have shown. Their words of support and encouragement carry a very special potency and confirm the importance of the royal role within the wider RNLI team.

Queen Victoria

The first female name ever to appear in the reports of the RNLI was Queen Victoria when she became Patron on her accession to the throne in 1837. True, some female subscribers had been recorded, but essentially for the first thirteen years of the RNLI's existence, anyone of significance was male.

Queen Victoria was enthusiastic about the cause, as was her husband, the Prince Consort. They both made financial contributions and encouraged foreign royalties to give their support. Queen Victoria herself funded two lifeboats. The first was from the estate of Samuel Fletcher, who died without a will in 1885. The estate having passed to the Queen through the Duchy of Lancaster, she gave part of the estate to the RNLI for the building of a new lifeboat for Blackpool, to be named *Samuel Fletcher of Manchester*. This lifeboat was replaced in 1896 by another lifeboat of the same name. Queen Victoria's gifts served Blackpool for a total of forty-four years.

In 1887, to coincide with the Queen's Golden Jubilee, the RNLI decided to build and maintain in perpetuity a lifeboat named after her. The first *Queen Victoria* was stationed at Bembridge and named by the Queen's daughter-in-law, the Duchess of Edinburgh.

Subsequent lifeboats of the same name were stationed at Porthoustock and St Peter Port, but after this no more carried her name.

Queen Victoria's generosity to the RNLI continued throughout her long reign. She had been its Patron for sixty-three years when she died in 1901, and by then was 'one of its largest annual subscribers'. From 1862, medals for gallantry carried the head of the Queen.

Queen Alexandra

Queen Victoria's eldest son, Edward, Prince of Wales became closely involved with the RNLI and his wife Alexandra supported his interest, becoming Vice Patron in 1883. At their home, Marlborough House, in 1884, she and her husband received Robert Egerton, coxswain of the Clacton-on-Sea lifeboat and Rowland Hughes, coxswain of Moelfre lifeboat. The Princess presented both with medals that had been awarded by the RNLI.

After her husband's death, Alexandra became Patron in 1913 and held this office until she died in 1925. The Freemasons funded three lifeboats and named them in her honour. They were all stationed at Hope Cove in Devon between 1878 and 1930.

Princess Louise, Duchess of Argyll

Enthusiasm for the lifeboat service was shared by another of Queen Victoria's children, the Princess Louise, Duchess of Argyll. Her first encounter was attending a naming ceremony for the lifeboat *Atherfield* on the Isle of Wight in 1891.

She travelled to Manchester in 1894 to receive purses from the Manchester and Salford Ladies of the Lifeboat Saturday Fund. Her most significant contribution came in 1923 when she became Patron of the newly formed Ladies' Lifeboat Guild. Her task was to inspire new members to even greater support for the lifeboat crews and her speech at the first conference sought out their empathy: '… no Institution can be nearer to the hearts of our women with more penetrating interest, love and sympathy …'.

Princess Louise led the Ladies' Lifeboat Guild from the front, visiting the Flag Day depots on more than one occasion and ensuring that guests (all 150 of them) at the meeting of the General Council in 1927 received a personal welcome from herself. Other RNLI fundraising events she attended include joining Queen Mary in 1922 at the showing of the Citroen film of the crossing of the Sahara Desert, and accompanying King George V, Queen Mary and the Prince of Wales in 1930 for the lifeboat variety matinee at the Hippodrome.

She was Patron of the Ladies' Lifeboat Guild until she died in 1939.

Princess Beatrice

The first RNLI engagement for the youngest of Queen Victoria's children, Princess Beatrice, was to open a fête in York in 1905. Her significant contribution was as Patron of the Isle of Wight Branch, a role she held for twenty-four years until her death in 1944.

Queen Mary

Queen Mary's husband, George V, had real maritime interests stemming from his service in the Royal Navy, and gave great service to the RNLI. He was strongly supported by his wife who, as Duchess of Cornwall and York, became President of the Ladies' Auxiliary of the Lifeboat Saturday Fund in 1895. In 1902, soon after becoming Princess of Wales, she became a Vice President of the RNLI and the following year received at Marlborough House ladies from all parts of the country who presented her with purses of money collected for the lifeboat service.

The first reference to a royal lady stepping on to a lifeboat occurs in 1909. Then, as Princess of Wales, Mary viewed the launch of Newquay lifeboat, down what was then the steepest slipway on the coast, and then went on board. She is renowned as a strong and stalwart lady and she and the King were anxious to show support and appreciation for the lifeboat service during the First World War.

When she died in 1953, she had given fifty-eight years of service to the RNLI.

Princess Mary

Third child of King George V and Queen Mary and their only daughter, Princess Mary had two lifeboats named after her. The first, *Princess Mary*, was stationed at Padstow in 1929, and the second, *Princess Royal*, entered service ten years later at Hartlepool.

Princess Mary was the most public-spirited member of the royal family, with her interests focusing on women's activities, including nursing and Girlguiding. Even so, she supported the family tradition and was active with the RNLI. She named four lifeboats: *Stanhope Smart* at Bridlington; *Herbert Joy the Second* at Scarborough in 1931; her own lifeboat, *Princess Royal* at Hartlepool in 1941; and finally, *City of Leeds* at Redcar in 1951.

Queen Elizabeth, the Queen Mother

When Lady Elizabeth Bowes-Lyon married the Duke of York in 1923, she may not have known that she was to start an association with the RNLI that was to last for the rest of her life – some eighty-one years.

The Duke was already a keen supporter, and her first RNLI engagement was to join him in touring the London Flag Day depots at Kensington, Fulham, the City and the West End in May 1924. It was the RNLI's centenary Flag Day, and a visit from the young royals was greatly appreciated by the volunteers. She was to make similar visits in 1931.

As Duchess of York, she accepted an invitation to name a lifeboat at Montrose in September 1926. She travelled there with her husband and her father, the Earl of Strathmore. The day had been designated a local holiday and 10,000 people gathered to see the Duchess release a bottle of Australian wine to smash on the bows of the lifeboat as she said the words: 'I name this boat the *John Russell*.'

The Duchess of York at the naming of the Montrose lifeboat *John Russell* in 1926.

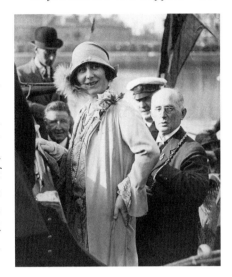

Loud cheers greeted the Duchess as she and her husband went afloat for a short tour of the docks. On coming ashore she was presented with a bouquet of flowers by a six-year-old girl, the granddaughter of Coxswain William Stephen. This was only the fourth time that a member of the royal family had named a lifeboat, and it was clearly felt to be a great honour that the Duchess had agreed to undertake the duty. George F. Shee, Secretary of the Institution, made a speech of warm thanks:

> Her Royal Highness is a daughter of the County of Forfar, and to-day she has come to link herself with the sea and with that service which is the finest flower of our dominion of the sea. By doing so she will strengthen the affection which all the people, not only of Forfarshire and of Scotland, but of Great Britain feel for her. In that part of Britain, south of the Tweed, which Scotland annexed long ago, there is a beautiful county which has earned the title of the ' Delectable Duchy.' There is another county of England, whose history is linked with the red Rose of Lancaster. But it has remained for Forfarshire to give to England and to Britain the Delectable Duchess, the white Rose of York. I offer you, Madam, the humble and cordial thanks of all present here today, and of those hundreds of thousands who throughout the British Isles honour and cherish the Life-boat Service, and I ask all present to express their thanks by giving three cheers for Her Royal Highness the Duchess of York.

The official account of the ceremony notes that cheers from the crowd punctuated the address, but on its conclusion 'The cheers were loud and prolonged, rushing in a growing volume of sound round the sides of the dock basin'. The celebrations continued into the evening with a grand firework display, which included portraits of the Duke and Duchess of York and the *John Russell*.

The Duchess must have enjoyed the experience because she would go on to name a further six lifeboats. At Arbroath in 1932 she named the *John and William Mudie* and again many thousands of people came to watch. This lifeboat went on to perform a wartime rescue of seven crew members of a bombed hopper barge, which became caught in the crossfire between German planes and British minesweepers in February 1940. One of the first messages of congratulations came to the coxswain from the lady who had named the lifeboat. She was now Queen Elizabeth and it was obvious that she cared about the crew.

King George VI consented to become Patron of the RNLI on his accession in 1937 and Queen Elizabeth agreed soon afterwards to do the same. Together they undertook a number of lifeboat station visits, but it was not until after the King had died that – now as Queen Elizabeth, the Queen Mother – she named another lifeboat in 1956. This was in

Scotland, at Thurso, where she named the thirty-first lifeboat to be donated to the RNLI by the Civil Service Lifeboat Fund. She named it *Dunnet Head (Civil Service No. 31)*. She returned in 1971 to name the next lifeboat for Thurso, *The Three Sisters*. After the ceremony she went afloat and took the wheel out in the Pentland Firth under the watchful eye of Coxswain Gilbert Reid.

Two other lifeboat namings took place in 1975 and 1979. Firstly at St Helier, where the Queen Mother named the *Thomas James King*. This was a special occasion because the lifeboat was named in honour of one of Jersey's most famous coxswains, Thomas King. In 1949 he led his crew to the very daring rescue of four men from a yacht in trouble in the pitch dark among dangerous rocks. For this bravery he was awarded the RNLI Gold Medal, but then the people of Jersey showed their admiration by raising the money for a new lifeboat to carry his name. Happily Thomas King, aged eighty-nine, was able to attend the ceremony, where his medal was formally presented and at which he had a lengthy conversation. On the following day, at Portsmouth, the Queen Mother attended a handing over ceremony for the new lifeboat for Walmer – a station she had visited in 1956 to present a vellum commemorating their centenary. Almost completely funded from within the county of Hampshire from an appeal launched by Sir Alec Rose, the renowned round-the-world yachtsman, the lifeboat was named *Hampshire Rose*.

The 1979 naming ceremony at Dover was marked by bad weather, which was unfortunate because it was attended by many members of rotary clubs who had travelled from all over the country for the naming of the lifeboat *Rotary Service*. Typically undaunted, she coped well with the persistent rain.

Understandably, the Queen Mother felt a particular closeness to the lifeboat stations in Scotland, and so it was that she shared the shock and distress of the loss of the Longhope lifeboat crew. On 17 March 1969, going to the aid of a Liberian cargo vessel *Irene*, the lifeboat was overwhelmed by mountainous seas and the lives of all eight crewmen were

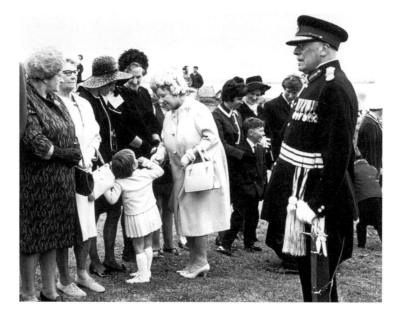

In 1970 the Queen Mother met the families of the lifeboat crew who lost their lives in the Longhope Lifeboat Disaster.

The Queen Mother at the naming of the Thurso lifeboat *The Queen Mother* in 1989.

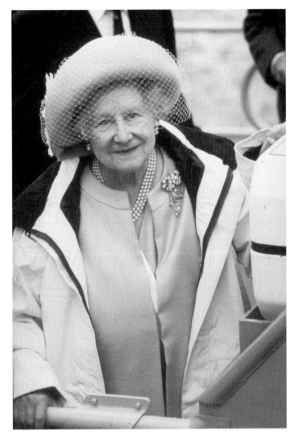

lost – a devastating tragedy for their families and the small community of Longhope on the island of Hoy.

Anxious to share her sympathy with the wives and relatives, hers was one of the first telegrams to arrive at Longhope. Just over a year later, she undertook the responsibility of unveiling a bronze statue erected in tribute to the brave men, in Osmondwall Cemetery, Orkney. She took time to speak personally with the widows and families before attending a memorial service in Walls Old Kirk where she unveiled a plaque recording the names of the eight lifeboat men. This is almost certainly the closest a member of the royal family has come to the harsh reality that lifeboat crews really do risk their own lives when they go to the aid of others in danger.

Queen Elizabeth the Queen Mother maintained a close relationship with Thurso Lifeboat Station, returning there in 1989 to undertake what transpired to be her last lifeboat naming. Very appropriately the lifeboat was named *The Queen Mother*. She was, as ever, warmly received, and by now she was affectionately known by the crew as 'wifie'. On this occasion she delighted everyone by donning the crew's yellow protective jacket and going on board the lifeboat. RNLI officials were understandably anxious about how the eighty-nine-year-old lady would cope, but cope she did – with aplomb! Coxswain William Farquhar, who was close to the royal guest throughout the trip, recalls that she was quite disappointed to have to go so slowly!

Long service and her very warm and personal approach to people can explain the affection the RNLI had for the Queen Mother. It also explains the enthusiasm to help celebrate her 100th birthday in 2000. An article in *The Lifeboat*, Autumn 2000, describes how the RNLI saluted the lady who had, by her 100th year, given seventy-six years' service to the cause of saving life at sea:

Lifeboat men and women from England, Wales, Scotland and Northern Ireland helped to make up the RNLI's contingent that took part in HM Queen Elizabeth the Queen Mother's

100th birthday parade on 19 July at Horseguards Parade, in London. The RNLI's colour party accompanied two contrasting lifeboats manned by the volunteers. The *Queen Victoria* is a restored pulling and sailing lifeboat from 1887, and was pulled by a team of horses. The *Miss Miriam and Miss Nellie Garbutt* is a modern Atlantic 75 rigid inflatable lifeboat, and is the fastest in the RNLI fleet with a top speed of 32 knots. Stormy Stan also joined in the parade, riding in his own vehicle.

Everyone agreed that the day was extremely enjoyable, and the RNLI was proud to be included in the celebrations. In the end everything ran smoothly, but that is not to say that there weren't some stressful moments in the preparation. The original plan included an all-weather Mersey class lifeboat instead of the Atlantic 75. It was only days before the parade that royal officials informed RNLI organisers that the Mersey was too tall. It would not fit under the special canopy that was being erected. Fortunately, as an emergency organisation, the RNLI is experienced at reacting quickly and the substitute Atlantic 75 was brought into service.

When the Queen Mother died in 2002, the feeling throughout the RNLI was that of sadness as a dear friend had been lost. The Chairman, Peter Nicholson, and the former coxswain of Thurso, William Farquhar, represented the RNLI at her funeral.

Princess Marina, Duchess of Kent

After her husband, the Duke of Kent, died on active service in 1942, the Duchess accepted the invitation to succeed him as President of the RNLI. She would go on to give almost twenty-six years' service to the Institution.

Quickly establishing her own special style, her first concern was to meet as many people as possible. This could not be done at a public meeting, as during war years the diary of the royal family was kept secret. The solution was a private tea party held at the Savoy Hotel in London, at which she could meet the Committee of Management, the City of London Branch and the Central London Women's Committee, as well as Life Governors and key employees. At this gathering she made a speech, stating: 'I look forward after the war to meeting the crews of the boats from many parts of the country, and to thanking them for their courageous deeds of mercy in these critical years.'

Wartime restrictions had made it impossible to hold the RNLI Annual Meeting at which awards for gallantry were made. In 1945, the first for six years was arranged, and it was the Duchess of Kent who presented the awards on this memorable occasion. She had a busy time, as exceptionally there were eight Gold Medals to present. They went to: Robert Cross, of the Humber, who won the Gold Medal twice, and also the Silver Medal, the Thanks on Vellum and the George Medal, having helped to rescue 244 lives; Henry Blogg GC BEM, of Cromer, who also won the Silver Medal twice, and the British Empire Medal, and helped to rescue 428 lives; Lieutenant William H. Bennisorf CGM, RNVR, of Hartlepool; John B. McLean, of Peterhead, who helped to rescue 414 lives; William Gammon of the Mumbles, who also won the Bronze Medal; Patrick Murphy, of Newcastle, Co. Down, who also won the Bronze Medal twice; and John Boyle of Arranmore, who also won the Dutch Gold Medal for gallantry in saving life. The Duchess of Kent also presented vellums to three

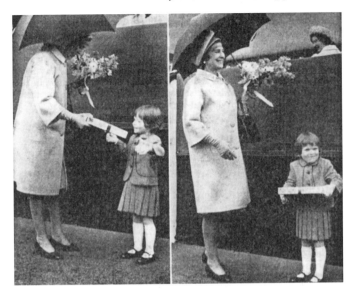

Princess Marina, Duchess of Kent presenting four-year-old Alison Gibb with a box of chocolates in return for the flowers just received from her. St Katharine Docks, London, 1966.

of the four RNLI Honorary Life Governors appointed during the war: Lady Florence Pery, of London; Councillor Mrs. F. M .H. Coleman, MBE, of Clacton-on-Sea; and Captain A. Stephen, of Fraserburgh.

Owing to illness, the Duchess was unable to attend the Annual Meeting in 1947. She had especially wanted to be there because among the awards were certificates to the widows of the crew of Mumbles Lifeboat Station who had lost their lives when the lifeboat capsized in a hurricane. She had to send her apologies, but her prepared speech was read out and included the words: 'With a heavy and understanding heart I pray that the families of these men may be comforted by the world-wide tributes to them ... We shall not forget them or their relatives.' She did not forget, for when she visited Swansea the following year for a festival of music, she met and spoke with the widows.

As with other members of the royal family, the Duchess accepted many invitations to name lifeboats. In the tribute given on behalf of the RNLI after her death in 1968, it was said by Captain Wyndham-Quin, RN:

Perhaps a naming ceremony on a fine day gave her the greatest pleasure, with the band playing, flags flying and a warm reception from the big crowds which were always present. The presentations and actual ceremony over, she would meet and talk with the wives of the crew and local officials, and many others connected with the branch. This she did with her own inimitable charm and humour, giving the greatest pleasure to all who were presented.

As well as attending fundraising dinner dances near to her home in London, she ensured she fulfilled her stated intention made in 1942 to meet and thank the brave crews, and so travelled extensively, covering: Bridlington★; Tynemouth★; New Brighton★; Margate★; Plymouth★; Padstow★; Fraserburgh★; Walton and Frinton★; Southend-on-Sea★; Stornoway★; Tenby★; Port St Mary★; Douglas★; Berwick-upon-Tweed★; Arbroath★; Barra Island★; Mallaig★; Newhaven★; Dundee★; Sheringham★; Shoreham★; Llandudno★;

St David's★; Cromer★; Wells★; Dover★; St Katherine Dock, London★; Sheringham; Weston-super-Mare; Ramsgate; Swansea (Mumbles); Penlee; Aberystwyth; Barmouth; Port Erin; Eyemouth; St Abbs; and Dunbar (places followed by ★ indicate naming ceremonies).

Her visit to the RNLI depot at Boreham Wood was welcomed by staff who demonstrated the rigging loft, machine shop and despatch department. The Duchess went home that day with a bell rope made in the rigging loft and a pair of brass candlesticks made in the machine shop.

Having presented so many medals as President of the RNLI, the Duchess was herself presented with a Gold Medal at a reception in 1967 held to mark her twenty-fifth year of service. It was given with the following words from the Chairman: 'I ask you, Madam, to accept from me this Gold Medal as a token of the esteem and respect and, if I may say it, the affection in which you are held by the whole service.'

The Duchess of Kent

The present Duchess of Kent has followed her predecessor in being a very keen supporter of the RNLI and a prodigious namer of lifeboats – sixteen in all. Formerly, as Katharine Worsley, she had an early introduction to lifeboats through family excursions and holidays on the Yorkshire coast. She would refer to the powerful impression these encounters made on her young mind in many of the speeches she made at RNLI events.

Her first public engagement for the RNLI was to accompany her husband, the Duke of Kent to the service in St Paul's Cathedral celebrating 150 years of the lifeboat service. Later in the same year she undertook her first naming of the lifeboat *Sir William Arnold* at St Peter Port. She must have been delighted to accept the invitation the following year to go to Whitby in her home county to name their new lifeboat *The White Rose of Yorkshire*. The Duchess drew the crowds and a happy picture of her on board was used for the cover of the next edition of *The Lifeboat* magazine. A firm bond was made with the lifeboat community of Whitby and the duchess would go on to name their next two lifeboats – *The City of Sheffield* in 1989, and *George and Mary Webb* in 1996. Her very last engagement for the

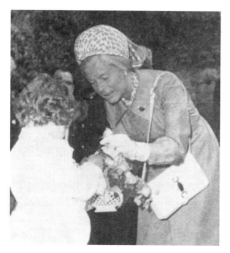

RNLI was at Whitby when she agreed to open the new boathouse in 2000.

The Duchess of Kent's ability to engage easily with people was much enjoyed at lifeboat stations and she gave generously of her time with the dreaded 'time schedule' often slipping back. It is a tradition at lifeboat stations to present a royal guest with flowers with the privilege going to a small child who is often quite daunted by

The Duchess of Kent takes out a rose from her bouquet and hands it back to five-year-old Susanne Gibbs, daughter of Coxswain Kenneth Gibb during a visit to Torbay Lifeboat Station in 1975.

all the attention. Early in her engagements the Duchess developed a practice of returning one flower from the bouquet to the child, which seemed to have the desired effect
of reducing the poor child's anxiety. On one occasion at Torbay, the Duchess was herself
presented with a lovely gift – two lobsters which had been caught by the deputy coxswain.

In 1975 and 1976 Plymouth and Ramsgate were both pleased to welcome her to name
their lifeboats, *Thomas Forehead and Mary Rowse* and *Ralph and Joy Swann*. Then in 1981,
the Duchess told everyone that she had 'jumped at the opportunity' to name the St Mary's
lifeboat *Robert Edgar*, having had such a happy holiday on the island earlier that year.

The Freemasons donated a lifeboat in 1982 to be named *Duchess of Kent*. As Grand
Master, the Duke of Kent handed over the lifeboat for his wife to perform the naming,
which she said was 'a singular honour'. Throughout the 1980s and 1990s the Duchess trav-
elled far and wide naming lifeboats at Exmouth (*Caroline Fish*), Alderney (*Foresters Future*),
Wells (*Doris M. Mann of Ampthill*), North Sunderland (*Grace Darling*), London Docklands
(*Marine Engineer*), Scarborough – where she was warmly welcomed 'back home' (*Fanny
Victoria Wilkinson and Frank Stubbs*), Anstruther (*Kingdom of Fife*), Berwick (*Joy and Charles
Beeby*), Silloth (*Spirit of Cumbria*), and Alderney (*Roy Barker 1*).

The Duchess of Kent's very personal touch and great concern for lifeboat people was
very clear when she presented the awards in 1987, 1990 and 1995. She spoke at some length
to each awardee and emphasised in her addresses her admiration for the courage of lifeboat
crews. As she had done in many of her naming ceremony speeches, she acknowledged the
great contribution made by the families: 'Lifeboat men's wives have to show their own sort
of quiet courage and forbearance whenever a boat is launched and I admire them deeply
for it.'

Royal visits bring a very particular challenge to RNLI staff who have the responsibility to ensure that all arrangements are impeccable and – most particularly – that the time
schedule (measured in minutes) is strictly adhered to. The author's own experience of this
going out of the window was on a tour of Cumbrian stations with the Duchess of Kent
in 1995. We were doing nicely and I could almost dare to relax when, between visits, the
royal car in front of the one I was travelling in with the Lifeboat Inspector suddenly took
an unscheduled turning to Penrith. Frantic phone calls from one car to the other revealed
that the Duchess had decided to go shopping – to the famous Toffee Shop in the town. It
seems that she had a particular liking for their fudge! We did make up the time later, but not
without many anxious moments.

Princess Alexandra

Princess Alexandra received a very warm welcome when she accompanied her mother,
Princess Marina, to the Annual Meeting in 1952. It was her first public appearance at a
formal meeting and the Chairman presented her with a silver lifeboat as a memento of
the occasion. Having been told by the young Princess that she had never been out in a
lifeboat, he promised to 'see that is remedied before too long. The Princess will find it
a very exhilarating experience to go out in a lifeboat, perhaps in a gale wind.' Her wish
was to be fulfilled many times in the years ahead as she became more and more involved

in the lifeboat service. She shared her mother's pleasure in naming lifeboats and it must have been a particular pleasure at her first ceremony at Wick in 1971 to name the lifeboat *Princess Marina*.

It was quite a family outing in 1973 when, accompanied by her husband, Sir Angus Ogilvy, and her mother-in-law, the Dowager Countess of Airlie, she named the Montrose lifeboat, *The Lady MacRobert*. The Dowager Countess was President of Montrose Ladies' Lifeboat Guild. Her daughter would come to the rescue in 1994 when Princess Alexandra had an accident preventing her from undertaking the naming at Arbroath. The countess named *Inchape* on behalf of her sister-in-law.

An unlikely place for the Princess to come across a lifeboat crew was Stockport, which she visited in 1974. Here, though, was an enthusiastic group of men called the Stockport Crew of Lifeboat Auxiliaries, and she noticed they were wearing red crew stocking hats. She told them that she had been given two for her children but one had been lost. Immediately one man whipped off his hat and offered it to her. With a smile she accepted.

Princess Alexandra accepted invitations to name four lifeboats in the 1980s. Each ceremony was very different. At Shoreham Harbour in 1981, she met the donor of *The Davys Family*, Mrs A. Mason, and said she felt certain that she would be proud of the work of her lifeboat and of the crew. Ten years later the Princess would be back at Shoreham Harbour to name *Hermione Lady Colwyn*. Naming the Stornoway lifeboat *Sir Max Aitken II* did not involve a long journey to Scotland. It was actually named near the home of Sir Max on the Isle of Wight in 1984.

Two years later, the Princess travelled to Tenby for an especially emotional ceremony. The lifeboat *Sir Galahad* had been largely funded by an appeal by the Royal Fleet Auxiliary in tribute to the men who lost their lives in the Falklands War. In acknowledgement of this, Princess Alexandra said:

> Your new lifeboat will open a fresh chapter in the station's history – her crew will carry on the proud traditions. She is named in memory of men who lost their lives serving others in

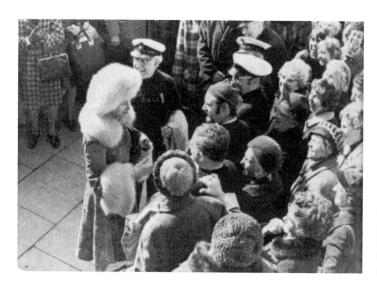

In 1974 Princess Alexandra accepts a red crew hat given by a member of Stockport Auxiliary Crew.

Princess Alexandra presenting the Individual Supporter of the Year Award 2006 to Chelsea Pensioner Sgt Bob Martin.

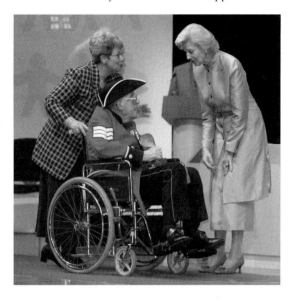

the Royal Fleet Auxiliary. It seems a most fitting tribute as this boat will also serve – in saving lives. Those who worked so hard in raising the money to provide the lifeboat must be proud to see her today and to think ahead to the work she will do in future years.

The welcome at Portpatrick when the Princess went to name *Mary Irene Millar* was so warm that her scheduled departure time went out the window. The Ladies' Guild had prepared such a splendid tea and there were so many lifeboat people to talk with, that she left a full hour later than had been intended. Some of the time had been taken up with her impromptu visit to the kitchen to thank the ladies working hard behind the scenes.

A similar delay to the schedule occurred at Penarth when, delighted to be reintroduced to a member of the Ladies' Guild she had formerly met, she chatted for so long that a diplomatic reminder of the time was made to her. Her response is remembered as being: 'When I was seventeen I realised I could either do what other people told me or do what I wanted. I chose the latter, so I think I'll just finish talking to everybody.'

'Talking to everybody' is a very good way to summarise the service given by Princess Alexandra, who must have had conversations with many hundreds of lifeboat people. Apart from all the naming ceremonies, she has made visits to lifeboat stations from as far away as Scarborough to St Peter Port, has visited the RNLI stand at the Boat Show in London, and very significantly has twice – in 1988 and 2006 – presented the awards to crew and volunteers. On each occasion it was noted how generous she was with her time for each individual.

Princess Margaret

Princess Margaret's association with the RNLI was quite slight until 1979 when she saved the day for Margate Lifeboat Station, and is remembered very kindly for doing so.

Her first contacts were a visit to St Peter Port in 1959 where she clearly enjoyed speaking with the crew there, and visits to the RNLI stand at the Boat Show in 1966 and 1972. The formal engagement at Margate was to name the lifeboat *Silver Jubilee (Civil Service No. 38)*, standing in at very short notice for Princess Alexandra who was unwell. It was a November day and the weather was particularly wretched, very cold with a thick blanket of fog. The Princess was delayed in arriving but all went well with the ceremony and sub-

At Margate Lifeboat Station in 1979, Princess Margaret is presented to the crew after naming their new lifeboat *Silver Jubilee (Civil Service No. 38)*.

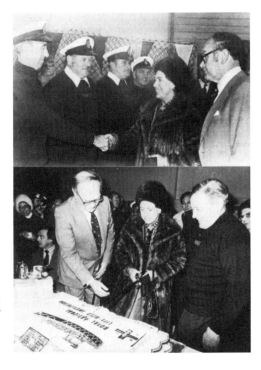

sequent inspection of the lifeboat. Princess Margaret wisely came attired in a warm fur coat. Before leaving in the ever thickening fog she had tea, which was rather special as a member of the crew was a master baker and had made a beautiful christening cake.

Princess of Wales

To commemorate the wedding of Prince Charles and Lady Diana Spencer in 1981, an appeal was launched with the aim of raising £100,000 for a new lifeboat in Wales. It was an ambitious target, but the organisers hoped that every town council, business organisation, sporting and sailing club would give their support. The appeal was successful, and the following year the Prince and Princess of Wales went to Barmouth where the new lifeboat would be stationed.

It was a cold November day, but the prospect of seeing the royal couple drew a large crowd and the sun obliged by coming out just as they arrived in the town. During the service of dedication hymns were sung in both languages and the Princess joined in with both. When she named the lifeboat *Princess of Wales* it was greeted with loud cheers. After some time talking with the coxswain and crew, the royal couple took their leave for another engagement – and the sun promptly disappeared!

A visit to Newlyn in 1987 to open the new fish market gave the Princess the opportunity to meet the crew of the Penlee lifeboat, and in the same year she performed one further lifeboat naming at Aith, the RNLI's most northerly lifeboat station. She named *Snolda* while Prince Charles had the task of opening the new lifeboat pier.

Princess Royal

Princess Anne had an exciting start to her relationship with the RNLI, joining her father and Prince Charles on a trip afloat a United States Coast-Guard cutter that had been loaned to the Institution for trials. Together they must have had fun in this fast forty-four-foot steel boat off the coast of Cowes in July 1974. The Princess enjoyed the sea and sailing – in future years this was to be reflected in her support for the RNLI.

Public duties in the West Country in the 1980s brought her visits to St Ives, Brixham and St Peter Port, but it was not until 1986 that – as Princess Anne – she had her first experience of naming a lifeboat. It was at Southend and the day started with her opening the new railway, which runs along the pier to where the lifeboat station is located. Her next task was to name the new lifeboat, which was to carry the name of a local hero, *Percy Garon*. He had been decorated in both World Wars and had been a member of the Southend Branch of the RNLI for forty-five years, many of them as Honorary Secretary.

Raymond Baxter, TV personality and member of the Committee of Management, welcomed the Princess with a speech laden with metaphor. He said how appropriate it was that Princess Anne should name the Atlantic 21, 'the only class of RNLI lifeboat controlled from what can only be described as a saddle, complete with stirrups, into which the feet are inserted – heels well down, of course – not only to ensure staying on board over the bigger jumps, but also to facilitate responsive control of immense power and outstandingly well bred performance, however demanding the course or the going.'

Princess Anne appears to have accepted all this with good humour, but did remark that she had been disappointed to learn that she would not have time for a trip on board the lifeboat, and even more so having seen it! Her desire was fulfilled the following year, though, when it was organised for her and her son, Peter Phillips, to have a trip afloat an identical lifeboat at Lymington. She had an enjoyable time and took the helm of the *Frank and Mary Atkinson* and came ashore to find a surprise – the donors of the lifeboat that carries their name were waiting alongside and presented the Princess with a cheque for £50,000 for the RNLI.

Five years later, now the Princess Royal, she returned to Southend to open the new boathouse and later that year undertook to bestow on the St Ives lifeboat her own name, *The Princess Royal (Civil Service No.41)*. The ceremony was followed by a trip round the bay with the Princess helming the lifeboat for most of the time.

Her boating skills and enthusiasm for going afloat prompted a request to her from the RNLI marketing department to endorse 'Offshore' the new class of membership for boat owners, which was being launched at the London Boat Show in 1997. She readily agreed, and subsequently became Offshore Member No. 1. The Princess referred to this when she presented the awards at the Barbican in 2000. In a speech that is still held to be one of the best made in recent years, she said that: 'As a yachtswoman and a member of the RNLI's "Offshore" scheme ("nobody twisted my arm") she had learned how quickly things can go wrong at sea.' She spoke of 'people like me who might take a boat out one day in

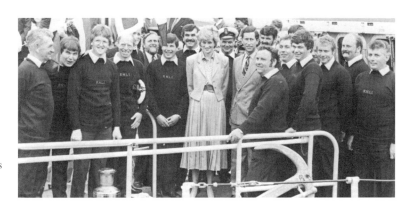

The Prince and Princess of Wales at Aith in 1986, where the Princess named their new lifeboat *Snolda*.

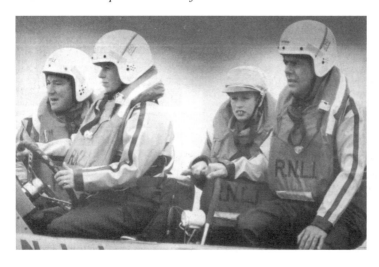

The Princess Royal with her son Peter Phillips on board Lymington's Atlantic 21 lifeboat in 1987.

unsuitable conditions, not having paid enough attention to the weather forecast', and who might then become an RNLI statistic. She continued:

> But in some ways I am only grateful people still go to sea and do enjoy the sea, who are prepared to take a few risks – I just wish that they would learn that there are some risks which you can prevent and avoid.

In 2007 the Princess Royal made a visit to the Lifeboat College to see for herself the training facilities that the Queen had opened. There was much discussion about the most appropriate scenario for the Bridge Simulator; a gentle sea had been programmed for Her Majesty but it was thought that the Princess would appreciate something rather more lively. Not so … the exercise had only been running for less than a minute when those in attendance outside heard her voice saying: 'If you don't tone that down immediately, I'm out of here!' The sea state was immediately reduced and all was well.

Queen Elizabeth II

Our present Queen's formal relationship with the RNLI began when in 1947 she made a donation of £180 – the balance of her wedding present from Kimberley in South Africa. The accompanying message said it came 'with her good wishes and those of the people of Kimberley'. The following year she sent a further cheque, this time from the royal wedding presents exhibition fund.

As Princess Elizabeth she made just one visit to a lifeboat station, St Helier in 1949, before the untimely death of her father in 1952 brought the responsibilities of the Crown, and with those, her agreement to be Patron of the RNLI.

Lifeboat communities threw themselves into the Queen's Coronation celebrations the following year and special events, including regattas, pantomimes, dances and parades were organised on the coast and by inland supporters. Four lifeboats took part in the Coronation

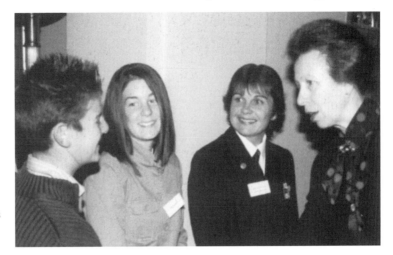

At the annual presentation of awards ceremony in 2005, the Princess Royal meets medallist Aileen Jones and her children, Frances and Dan.

Review of the Fleet in the Solent and the crews are recorded as giving three rousing cheers for Her Majesty as she passed by them on HMS *Surprise*.

A second Review of the Fleet in 1977 to commemorate her Silver Jubilee had just three lifeboats, but they were crammed with the best crew the RNLI could muster – twenty-three men, three with the British Empire Medal, eight with Silver Medals and sixteen with Bronze Medals for gallantry. It was obviously a great party, as afterwards one of the crew said: 'It's been marvellous. I hope I meet all these boys again … couldn't we do this every year?'

The Queen took the opportunity of her extensive travels throughout the country to visit lifeboat stations, including Yarmouth, Isle of Wight in 1965, St Peter Port in 1978, and Lerwick in 1981. On each occasion she spoke with the crews, taking an interest in their lifeboats, recent rescues and what they did for a living. History was made when the Queen named the Hartlepool lifeboat *The Scout* in 1977. This was the first time a reigning monarch had named a lifeboat, and how appropriate that it had been provided by the Scout Association, of whom she is also Patron. Over 1,500 scouts attended and were relieved that the unpleasant rain stopped and the sun came out just as the royal party arrived. After the ceremony the Queen inspected the lifeboat and spent time talking with crew wives and members of the Ladies' Guild.

The news that all the crew of Penlee had been lost on service brought an immediate telegram from the Queen:

> Prince Philip and I have heard with great regret the tragic news of the loss of the Penlee life-boat and her crew. I would like to record our admiration for their bravery and self-sacrifice. Please convey a message of deepest sympathy to their families.

When she visited Fraserburgh in 1992 she was presented with a cheque for £305,613, which was the proceeds from the Police Appeal, launched in celebration of her fortieth year on the throne. This money would be used to provide an all-weather lifeboat to be named *Her Majesty the Queen*. It would be placed in the RNLI Relief Fleet to serve all

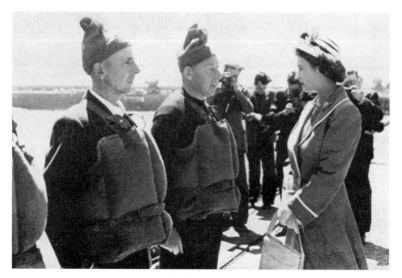

Princess Elizabeth meets members of St Helier crew on a visit to Jersey in 1949.

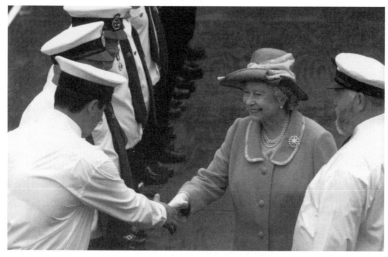

In 2003 HRH the Queen meets members of Plymouth lifeboat crew after she named their new lifeboat *Sybil Mullen Glover*.

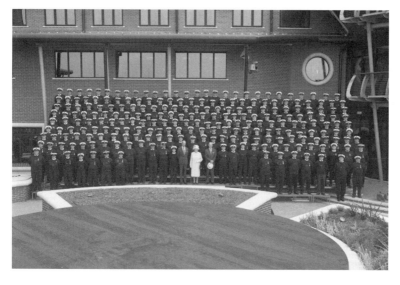

HRH the Queen at the opening of the Lifeboat College in 2004.

around our coast. In 1993 at Ramsgate, the Queen named 'her' lifeboat – and the sun was again shining.

She has since named two more lifeboats. The first was the Falmouth lifeboat *Richard Cox Scott* in 2002. This must have felt like quite a family day for Her Majesty, for, while taking a short trip afloat after the ceremony, she passed the sail training vessel *Prince William*, and then disembarked the lifeboat at Prince of Wales pier! The Queen met members of the family of Ruth Marygold Dix Scott, whose legacy had principally funded the lifeboat.

The weather was not so kind when she named the Plymouth lifeboat *Sybil Mullen Glover* in 2003. That was a very rainy day …

This lifeboat was principally funded from the legacy of Daphne Sybil Glover, a local distinguished marine artist.

The power of the monarch to bring together the RNLI community is demonstrated by two major events attended by the Queen. A special Buckingham Palace Garden Party to celebrate the 150th anniversary of the RNLI was hosted by the Queen on 16 July 1974. Hundreds of people from all over the country attended – probably it was the largest ever gathering of lifeboat supporters at one time and in one place. You were fortunate to be selected as a representative, as so many people wanted to attend.

On 28 July 2004, at the opening of the Lifeboat College in Poole, the Queen was greeted by the amazing sight of 233 coxswains and senior helms – one from every RNLI lifeboat station – lined up and awaiting the photograph that was to be taken of them with her and the Duke of Edinburgh. This was the first time in the 180-year history of the RNLI that a representative of every station had been in the same place at the same time. It was some feat of organisation and it was gratifying that the Patron was visibly impressed.

The Queen had already fulfilled two other official engagements in Dorset before arriving at the College. Her tour of the new facilities was quite arduous and included going afloat in the Bridge Simulator, as well as viewing a capsize demonstration in the Survival Pool. Sensitivity to Her Majesty's well-being ensured that the sea conditions in the Simulator were set as slight, but the waves in the Survival Pool were pretty lively! She waited patiently for the crew to return to the surface from underneath the upturned lifeboat. She asked John Allen, the then Inshore Lifeboat Training Manager, why they were taking so long. John was wondering just the same and recalls fabricating a convincing answer. What he did not know was that one of the team had shed his visor as the boat went over and under the boat all hands were frantically trying to put it back on before emerging!

After the ceremony, the royal party left aboard the new lifeboat for Castletownbere – the coxswain and crew had been training all week at the College. It was the first time that the Queen had visited RNLI Headquarters and her lively interest and support for what was a major new chapter in the story of the RNLI were encouraging to everyone: 'Having just seen some of the excellent training that is already being delivered, I am certain that the Lifeboat College will play a vital role in helping the RNLI to save even more lives.'

eight

WOMEN MOVING FORWARD

Forward from where to where?

From their earliest role using physical strength and stamina to move lifeboats in and out of the water, an absolutely vital but little recognised contribution to saving lives at sea …
To undertaking senior roles both in the local management of lifeboat stations and in the national governance, management and development of one of the largest and most respected charities in the UK and the Republic of Ireland.

Operationally, the extent of female contribution to the RNLI is certainly becoming less 'hidden' as more and more women volunteer for lifeboat crews and lifeguard teams. Also developing steadily has been a parallel process of women coming forward either as volunteers or as employees for roles which once were 'men only'. Nationally, women are now contributing at all levels within the organisation, the Board of Trustees and the Executive Team. Women are currently employed at senior levels in all Headquarters departments representing a broad range of professional expertise.

From a comparatively slow start, the RNLI has recognised the value of engaging more widely the skills and talents of women. The experience, perceptions and aspirations they bring to the organisation are extremely diverse. Speak to the individuals, though, and a common theme emerges. The modern women of the RNLI clearly see the value of saving lives at sea and want to help to do that as well as take their place in developing the efficiency and effectiveness of this voluntary and independent organisation.

Early pioneers

There were exceptions! Some women found themselves undertaking responsible roles normally held by men at lifeboat stations. It appears this mostly happened by default in unusual circumstances. Ahead of their time, these women were strong characters – operating in almost exclusively male environments, they had to have exceptional qualities.

Jane Hay of St Abbs Lifeboat Station.

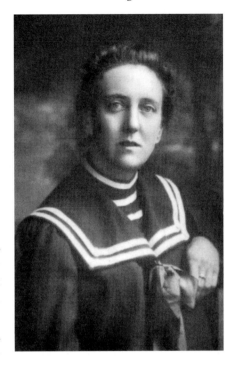

Jane Hay, Station Honorary Secretary, St Abbs, 1911–1914

Jane Hay had a short life – just fifty years – but one she filled with giving help to others. In St Abbs she is remembered as a woman with a big heart, but even bigger determination. She was their first Station Honorary Secretary and one of the first women in the RNLI to hold that position – possibly the first.

Her intention was to become a doctor, and while studying at London University she became interested in social work in the East End. Her health was not good and she was forced to terminate her studies and go to recuperate in the south of France. Once recovered, she returned to Edinburgh where all her energies were committed to social work, particularly on behalf of working girls and children. After a period in Turkey and Greece undertaking relief work following the Greco-Turkish war, her health was again a cause for concern and so she moved south to St Abbs and built a house overlooking the sea.

In this new environment, Jane became interested in the fishing families who she saw had hard lives and limited opportunities. She organised a club where those who wanted could learn new skills and enjoy social activities and arranged for the fishermen to have lessons in navigation. Her interest in sea rescue grew and she organised a children's rocket lifesaving brigade. They were issued with miniature equipment and had weekly exercises.

It was her experience in 1907, of watching a Danish ship, the *Alfred Erlandsen*, sink with all hands drowned, that persuaded her that St Abbs must have a lifeboat. Jane stood on the beach shouting out to the men that help was on its way, but it did not come in time – the nearest lifeboat was at Eyemouth, too far away. She campaigned for a lifeboat to be stationed at St Abbs and was successful. Eventually in 1911, with a new boathouse that Jane contributed £200 towards, and a new lifeboat, her efforts were fulfilled. She was appointed as Station Honorary Secretary with responsibilities to administer the station and to authorise launching the lifeboat when needed.

She was their Station Honorary Secretary for only four years before her sudden death, but her contribution was so much greater than the short period might suggest. In 1965, to honour her, it was decided to call the new lifeboat *Jane Hay*. In pride of place in the present lifeboat station is a picture of Jane – an acknowledgement of her outstanding commitment both to the cause of saving lives at sea and to St Abbs. What an amazing contribution this pioneering woman has made to the RNLI.

Letitia French of Palling Lifeboat Station in 1927.

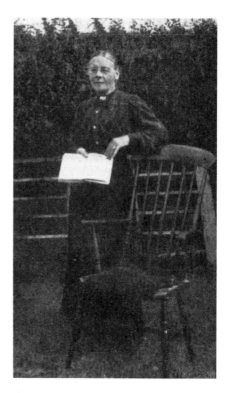

Letitia French, Station Honorary Secretary Palling, 1904–1928

In 1927 in one of a series of articles about 'Honorary Workers of the Institution', it was recorded in *The Lifeboat* that the only lifeboat station to have a woman Station Honorary Secretary was Palling in Norfolk. Letitia French took over this role from her father, Edward French, when he died in 1904, aged eighty. He had served the RNLI for thirty-eight years. In fact, he had been unwell for several years prior to his death, and during that time his daughter had taken over virtually all his responsibilities.

The author of the article may have had some difficulty in persuading Letitia to be interviewed. It seems she was a modest person and requested that the article should be devoted to her father's work and not her own. This was honoured, but her picture was included and the author slipped in at the end that in 1915 Letitia French was presented with a barometer with an inscription recording her service and the thanks of the RNLI.

Letitia died in 1928, and Palling Lifeboat Station was closed in 1930.

Marie Hoy, Station Honorary Secretary, Clogher Head, 1962–1981

When her husband died suddenly in 1962, Marie Hoy was asked by the Lifeboat Inspector if she could help the RNLI by temporarily taking on his role of Station Honorary Secretary of Clogher Head Lifeboat Station until another man was found. She agreed, but 'temporary' became permanent the following year after she had demonstrated how well she could do the job and she was asked to stay on. She continued in the role for nineteen years.

As wife of the Station Honorary Secretary, Marie had been actively involved in fundraising for the lifeboat service and decided to continue this alongside new operational responsibilities. She raised funds through appeal letters to individuals and businesses, but her main activity was organising Flag Days. Traditionally collections were made near the beach and the harbour, but Marie had the great idea of positioning collectors – and often it was members of the crew who helped with this – at all the church gates in Clogher Head and adjoining parishes. Her tactic was to catch people on their way into church when they felt more generous!

She explained away the ease with which she took over the responsibilities of Station Honorary Secretary from her husband. She said it was because she had been in close contact with the job while he had done it. She was being modest, because as well as a being a good organiser, she was a good people manager and knew how to nurture the support of others. She was strong and firm – qualities admired by the crew, who respected her immensely.

The lifeboat was called out less frequently in those days than now, and mostly to fishing boats. During Marie Hoy's time at Clogher Head, there was just one direct telephone line. It went into her house and was then transmitted to the boathouse and the mechanic's house by small switchboxes and extensions – a far cry from the technology of today, but the simple arrangement worked nonetheless.

For someone who had been asked to help out for a short while, Marie Hoy exceeded expectations by giving outstanding services to the RNLI in a role previously only held by men in her community. She retired in 1981, aged seventy-six, and was presented with the RNLI Gold Badge by Princess Alice the following year.

Dr Margaret Shimmin, Station Branch Chairman and Station Medical Officer, Aith, 1973–1884

When Margaret Shimmin and her husband moved to Aith in the early 1970s for her to be the GP for Bixter, she agreed to take on the role of Honorary Medical Adviser for Aith Lifeboat Station. It was not without some trepidation, as lifeboat services at this most northerly lifeboat station are often in the most wild and challenging conditions, and Margaret had little experience of the sea. Knowledge that her predecessors had fulfilled this role persuaded her to say yes, but she was uncertain about how she would be accepted by the all male crew.

Margaret soon showed a fearless approach when called out on a couple of occasions in the middle of the night to go with the lifeboat so that sick and injured seamen could receive emergency medical treatment. In rough seas and in the pitch dark she climbed from the lifeboat to the boat where the patient lay needing her help. The lifeboat crew was impressed with this doctor who made no fuss and simply got on with the job. It was a varied and demanding job too; there were times when she was called upon to go with the lifeboat to one of the many offshore islands where a sick person needed treatment or transfer to hospital. On other occasions she had to practise winch lifts from the lifeboat to search and rescue helicopter.

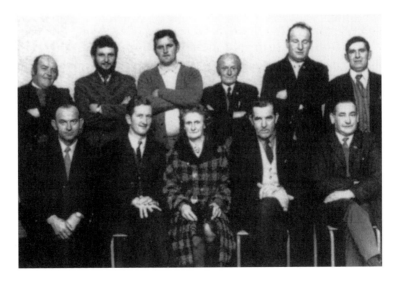

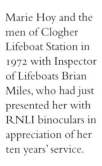

Marie Hoy and the men of Clogher Lifeboat Station in 1972 with Inspector of Lifeboats Brian Miles, who had just presented her with RNLI binoculars in appreciation of her ten years' service.

Margaret Shimmin on board the Aith lifeboat *Snolda* with Coxswain Hylton Henry in 1986.

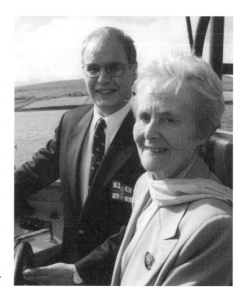

In fact, this attitude was entirely consistent with Margaret's personality and beliefs. She was very confident she could do any job that a man could do and actually did not like her gender referred to. Her excellent organisational skills were quickly recognised and she was asked to be the Station Branch Chairman. In this role she is remembered as being 'gently persuasive and consequently getting the best out of volunteers, delicately squeezing the last bit of effort out of everyone'. She added a third role when she took on the role of President of the Ladies' Lifeboat Guild.

Her special qualities were needed when, in 1986, Aith received not only a new lifeboat, *Snolda*, but also had major engineering and construction work for a new pier and boathouse. Margaret placed herself at the heart of the operations and her smiles and good nature oiled the wheels of progress. On completion of the work, she proposed that the RNLI invite a member of the royal family to the naming and opening ceremony. As ever, her powers of persuasion worked well and the Prince and Princess of Wales came to Shetland for the event. In Aith, it is remembered as a most memorable day, not least because Margaret, who by now had become 'a one person powerhouse' of organisation, had implemented the perfect plan.

Ten years later, by now retired and living in Wales, Margaret was the first choice of the lifeboat community in Aith to name their next lifeboat, *Charles Lidbury* – a happy reunion with her many friends. Margaret died in 2005 and will always be remembered in Aith for her enthusiasm for the RNLI, her sheer hard work for the lifeboat station and her achievement as a woman who insisted that her gender was irrelevant.

Zena Burslam, Station Chairman, Blackpool, 1989–2001

Zena Burslam took over the role of Station Chairman from her husband, Philip, after he died in 1989. It was not something she chose to do, but she was asked by the station committee. At first she declined, but then realising the relevance of the extensive committee experience she had both in the Ladies' Lifeboat Guild and in other organisations, she accepted. She took on the role at an important time for Blackpool Lifeboat Station, as it was expanding significantly as an inshore station.

Some years previously, a review of the deployment of lifeboats along the Fylde coast had recommended that Blackpool should become an inshore lifeboat station instead of an all-weather station. The case for this change was based on the high, and ever increasing, volume of incidents close to the beach to which the lifeboat crew was called out. Inshore lifeboats are quicker to launch and designed to operate in these shallower waters. After operating an all-weather lifeboat service since 1864, the Blackpool lifeboat community was unhappy about the proposed changes and appealed against it. The RNLI held to its decision and within the space of years Blackpool went from operating one to three inshore lifeboats.

Zena's clear intention was to support the crew and all the station volunteers through these changes, while continuing her own support for the Ladies' Lifeboat Guild and the Luncheon Club, both of which she had been actively involved with for many years. A further development came with the proposal to find bigger and better premises for the station, which after sixty years was no longer fit for purpose. A new building, which incorporated a visitor centre to take advantage of promoting the work of the RNLI to Blackpool's many thousands of tourists, was opened in 1998.

Zena looks back on her time as Station Chairman and recalls a mix of experiences. There were times when she felt it was definitely tough to be a woman in the role – so strong was the male culture at headquarters that she thinks it was not difficult to exclude her from some of the communications. Her experience locally was one that brought many satisfactions and pleasures – in fact her whole experience of the RNLI added a new dimension to her life and gave it greater purpose. Zena feels privileged to have witnessed at first-hand the bravery and total commitment of the crews, and she felt proud to see her son, John, join the crew.

Rowland Derbyshire, the current Lifeboat Operations Manager at Blackpool, is very certain that she has a special place in the history of the lifeboat station:

> Zena will always be remembered for her fierce devotion to the interests of the Blackpool station in general and the safety and welfare of the crew in particular. In her dealings with headquarters she managed to combine charm and courtesy with a dogged determination to accept nothing but the best for Blackpool. She bravely took on the job of Chairman after her husband died in office. By her work in that position and by her tireless fundraising efforts she gained the affection and respect of everyone at the station.

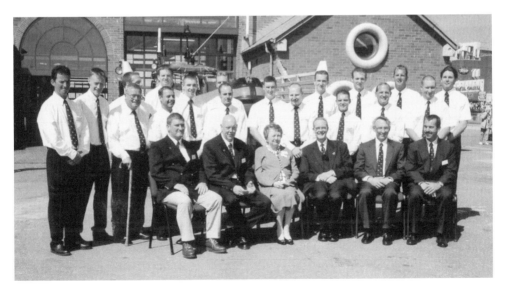

Zena Burslam with the men of Blackpool Lifeboat Station.

Lifeboat Operations Managers

In 2003 in an initiative to increase local responsibility for the management of lifeboat stations, the role of Station Honorary Secretary was discontinued and replaced by the Lifeboat Operations Manager. This is the senior operational volunteer at each lifeboat station and they carry significant responsibilities. Compared with the Station Honorary Secretary role, which dates back to the early days of the RNLI, the Lifeboat Operations Manager role carries higher levels of responsibility by placing more emphasis on the local management of the station and volunteers. There is still the significant responsibility of authorising the launch of the station lifeboat when it has been requested.

There are four women currently holding this important and responsible role – at Filey, Appledore and Douglas Lifeboat Stations they are volunteers. The Station Manager at Tower Lifeboat Station on the River Thames, where operational requirements are very different, is an RNLI employee.

Jo Ward, Lifeboat Operations Manager, Filey

The discussion is one that thousands of young couples have every time a marriage is planned: 'what date shall we have the wedding?' For Jo the discussion was cut short by her groom to be, John, stating quite adamantly that the date that had seemed best to her was quite impossible: 'We can't marry on that date – its Lifeboat Day!' So it was that another date was found.

John is a member of Filey lifeboat crew and would not dream of missing Lifeboat Day, but then Jo would not either. Her family connections to the RNLI are extensive; her father, who as a Trinity House Pilot in Amble, was involved with the lifeboat station there and then became a Deputy Launching Authority when he moved to Scarborough. Her godfather served on the lifeboat crew at Whitby, and was the inspiration for the lead character in the book *Three Fevers* by Leo Walmsley. It is a lifeboat tradition that Jo, who works in the office of the local school and has two children aged thirteen and eleven, has more than upheld herself.

She was the first woman ever to be appointed to the role of Lifeboat Operations Manager. When the previous Lifeboat Operations Manager stepped down, Jo was already actively involved with the station as the Station Administration Officer, and also as a member of the Ladies' Guild. She had a private thought that she 'would like to have a go at that', but dismissed it quickly, realising that she was very different to the traditional choice of a person for the role, who as a first requirement would be male. John, her husband, nurtured the idea and took quiet soundings at the station, which were positive. After this Jo was approached by the Station Chairman to apply. The crew was surprised but they were still positive. Jo is not entirely sure she was responsible for that reaction, preferring to think it was because John was such a respected member of the crew.

At her interview with the Deputy Lifeboat Inspector she gave the reasons why she thought she had the credentials; she had done service in the naval reserve, she is a competent sailor, she has a long association with the RNLI, '… and I am a mum who can bang heads together!' She got the job and was appointed on 1 February 2005.

Her memories of the early days are of realising that she had to quickly establish exactly what the responsibility of volunteering for a lifeboat crew actually meant. She was quite clear that it meant a commitment to training and updating knowledge and skills as well as turning up for shouts – for her, there was no question of picking and choosing. She recalls there was dissent but it was something she had to learn to manage because this was the way she wanted things to be done. She knew that she could not have people who would be a liability. 'Sometimes it was like walking on eggshells. Diplomacy skills are essential – I spent a lot of time sowing seeds in minds, hoping they would eventually take hold as their own idea. I think that has worked.' At the same time she was at pains to demonstrate to the volunteers that she was supporting them as best she could. Jo firmly believes that she is an integral part of a team that puts a lot of effort into saving lives, and like other members of the team, she has a specific set of responsibilities.

Not long after she started she had a very challenging day when they had three launches in the space of an hour. Jo recalls the day well:

> The station lifeboat, *Keep Fit Association*, had just returned from refit in Lymington. Almost as soon as the relief lifeboat, *Bingo Lifeline*, left Filey to return to a boatyard, the pagers went for a fishing boat in need of assistance to the south of Filey. We launched *Keep Fit* immediately with the original passage crew – unwashed, unshaved and unfed! Less than ten minutes later the pagers went again – this time for a holiday maker who had fallen on Filey Brigg and broken his leg. The paramedics requested the assistance of the ILB to evacuate the casualty to the awaiting ambulance. Meanwhile, *Bingo Lifeline* was being tasked to a job while on passage.

It was a complicated situation that required clear thinking and decisiveness, but Jo was able to find the right solutions and at the end of the day she realised that it had been a good job well done. She gets a similar feeling of satisfaction whenever she sees the lifeboat returning after a shout, knowing that her team have done well.

With a sea-going crew of thirty and a shore crew of eight, it is a strong team that she has at Filey. There is a good mix of ages and there are also four female crew members. Jo is confident that the right women come forward, but knowing what inner strength they need to possess, she does not actively campaign for female members. It will surely happen because the whole community in Filey are so support- ive of their lifeboat.

The floods in August 2002 and July 2007 presented the perfect opportunities for the lifeboat crew to provide a much-needed service for the people of the town. Using the coxswain's car to tow the inshore lifeboat on its trailer, they were first on the scene for some elderly residents whose bungalows were flooded. 'It's good to know you can help when the town has supported us for so many years', says Jo.

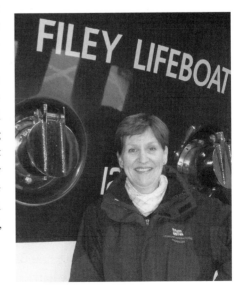

Jo Ward in the boathouse at Filey.

Wendy Dale, Lifeboat Operations Manager, Appledore

Wendy Dale and her husband made a conscious choice to make Appledore their home after a 'time out' period of travel around the UK: 'We saw the estuary and just knew it was the place for us.'

With a successful career behind her, Wendy wanted to make a complete lifestyle change. She wanted to make good use of the skills she had honed in very diverse roles in the private and voluntary sectors, by making a meaningful contribution within her new community. But why the RNLI? Born in Cornwall, Wendy recalls being taken to St Ives Lifeboat Station by her father and being told firmly that she could put money in the box, but she was *not* to go in the boathouse near the lifeboat – to this day she is not quite sure why. Then, as with many Cornish children, the memory of the Penlee disaster is seared into her memory. So the idea of joining the Appledore Ladies' Guild seemed like a good one. That was until the ladies informed her that they really did not want anyone to help with administration, thank you, and why not speak to the lifeboat station? Fine, thought Wendy, only to be told by the station that they did not need her either, thank you, and why not speak to the Ladies' Guild?

This 'ping pong' did not deter Wendy, who when Appledore Regatta came around volunteered to sell raffle tickets for the Ladies' Guild, and when they accepted her offer, she so excelled at the task that the Guild President made it known she wanted this person on the committee. After six months in the guild she was telephoned by the Station Honorary Secretary asking her if she would attend an interview for the Lifeboat Administration Officer post. It transpired that she was offered and accepted the position. Now she had a voluntary role with both the ladies and the men.

'In the guild I was happy to be behind the scenes. The guild makes much of its income from good quality home-cooked food events – cooking is enjoyable but using my other skills was preferable,' Wendy explains. At the station the administration role was a breeze for someone with all the corporate and management experience she had. There was a real challenge, though: 'I had to go carefully and thoughtfully to build their trust in me. I could see there were things that could be done differently and sometimes better, but to be seen to be too forceful would have been disastrous.' It was a careful process, but eventually Wendy was allowed to do things and so she knew that she was definitely establishing herself.

Becoming the Lifeboat Operations Manager was certainly not something that she anticipated or even aspired to, but after a period of a year without a person in the post she started to receive some mixed messages. Some spoke of the crew wanting her to take the role, others said that she would be too easily manipulated by the crew. At this time, Wendy was uncertain of what to do and initially offered to become a Deputy Launching Authority, which she did for several months before agreeing to take on the role of Lifeboat Operations Manager. This was prompted by her feeling that it was just not fair on the crew to have no one in this key position. She was encouraged by her husband, but made the provision there would be times in the summer months when she would be away sailing. This was understood and agreed to by the RNLI.

What followed for Wendy was a steep change in her levels of involvement and, more importantly for her, responsibility. Almost immediately there were senior administrative irregularities that had to be sorted, and suddenly she felt alone and very uncertain of where

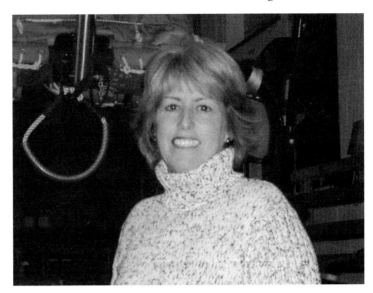

Wendy Dale in the
boathouse at Appledore.

the support for her lay. At the same time she was asked if she would take on chairmanship of
the guild and she accepted, seeing the real advantages of the operational and the fundraising functions becoming closer and feeling that under her she could lead such a movement.
A major aspiration was to make the work of the station better known and understood in
Appledore: 'We needed to open our doors, answer the questions, and be much more recep-
tive and available. I really believe that our community and the general public have a right
to this.'

In this she had the support of the coxswain and crew and they worked together to rein-
state the Open Days, and as well as the Sea Sunday service they organised a carol concert
in the boathouse. Wendy goes out and about giving talks to community groups and always
makes sure that she includes an invitation to visit the station. She makes the offer of organising photo-calls for cheque presentations, goes out to local fundraising events and believes
that the measurable increase in local donations is a consequence of the new 'open door'
approach.

The change of emphasis from administration to management that differentiates a Station
Honorary Secretary from a Lifeboat Operations Manager has had an impact virtually everywhere in the RNLI. Wendy was appointed with a Lifeboat Operations Manager job
description and has worked to deliver that; in particular, she has taken on improving the
quality of welcome to new crew volunteers, having observed that it was not done well at
the station – it was neither an easy message for her to deliver nor for the crew to receive.
Confident that it had to be better managed, mentors are now assigned to guide new volunteers and more supportive practices have been introduced. She has clear ideas about
how she and all station volunteers should present themselves in the local community, and is
prepared to stand her ground when necessary.

Wendy reflects that taking on the Lifeboat Operations Manager role was not the easiest
decision she ever made, and in the early days the job was far from easy. 'I was determined
to make it work – I was not going to give up. Gradually things got better and we moved

forward to a more professional approach. It took time and mutual confidence was built by a brick by brick process.' Paradoxically, as is so often the case in management roles, while surrounded by people, it can be lonely: 'There are no thanks – you have to do it because you believe it is the right thing to do.'

And on being a woman in this role? Wendy acknowledges that because women look at things differently, she cannot always anticipate how the men will react to some things and this can make for some interesting happenings, but with absolute certainty in her voice she says: 'When you know what you are doing and you can argue from an informed position, being a woman makes no difference.' The female skill of building and extending relationships is evidenced in what Wendy Dale has achieved as a Lifeboat Operations Manager and Chairman of the Ladies' Lifeboat Guild. She has enjoyed doing this and is proud to be in a position to be able to do things for the best interests of the RNLI and the community. Her 'to do' list is not finished yet – believing that the general public need to understand better the consequences of their actions, she wants to find ways to help in the prevention work of the RNLI.

Mary Corran, Lifeboat Operations Manager, Douglas

Douglas Lifeboat Station has always had a special place in RNLI history, as it was here that Sir William Hillary, founder of the RNLI, served as a member of the crew. The accounts of his personal bravery certainly confirm that he was a man who practised what he preached. It is not surprising that the people of Douglas have a great pride both in the unique history of their lifeboat station, and in all that the present crew achieve in saving lives in the difficult waters of the Irish Sea.

Mary Corran made her own contribution to Isle of Man history when she was appointed as Lifeboat Operations Manager in 2006 – the first woman on the island to hold the position. No one could be more proud of her achievement than her husband, Robert Corran, who retired as coxswain just three years earlier after thirty-nine years on the crew. Mary's family had no connection with the sea, but the Corrans have been fishermen for generations. She was keen to learn and readily confirms that Robert has taught her all she knows about the sea, the coast and boats – knowledge that is essential for her to manage the lifeboat station with competence.

When Mary and Robert married, she had little involvement with the station because of the tradition in Douglas that women did not go into the boathouse. Robert's father, William, was on the crew and acted as coxswain for some years. In the early days, Mary admits that she did not really feel much anxiety when her husband went out on a shout. When Robert became second coxswain, a telephone was installed at home and Mary became involved in helping to contact the crew when a lifeboat launch was required. She remembers that her awareness of the dangers the men faced also grew with the increase in her husband's responsibilities on board the lifeboat. Robert became coxswain in 1976, taking over from his cousin, Jack Griffiths.

Sometimes she would take their two small boys in the car to see the lifeboat launch or return. Douglas is a traditional slipway station so it was exciting for the children. It was also another small step in becoming involved, as well as helping influence her elder son, Brendan, to join the crew when he was old enough – he would go on to serve for twenty years. Gradually the old tradition of no women in the boathouse faded, and by 1990 Mary was giving a lot of welcome support to the Station Honorary Secretary, which culminated in a request in 2000 for her to take on the role of Deputy Launching Authority. This meant that Mary would be responsible for authorising the launch of the lifeboat in the absence of the Station Honorary Secretary – an extremely responsible task and a sure sign that Mary's ability had been recognised.

Appointment as Lifeboat Operations Manager came in 2006. Mary recalls that it was not entirely unexpected, as it had been mentioned to her some years previously, but she was still surprised because she did not think a woman would stand a chance. Confirmation came in a letter from the RNLI Chief Executive. Mary recalls it being no big surprise at the lifeboat station. With her long experience as coxswain's wife and Deputy Launching Authority, most people thought 'it was on the cards'. The reaction from others has been somewhat different – a number of people have been really surprised that a woman could do the job, but some have expressed genuine pleasure. Mary sees herself as a key ambassador for the organisation and is active in her community, giving talks about the RNLI, ensuring that all donations receive her personal thanks, and that the work of the crew receives good publicity.

In answer to the question what is good and what is not so good about this role, Mary immediately focuses on the feeling she has when she sees the lifeboat and crew return from a good service: 'It is good to see them all home safe and great to know that we have been able to help someone in trouble. Then I feel what an honour it is to be involved.' The 'not so good' answer is rather predictable: 'Paperwork!' Then with a gleam in her eye she says: 'And also when I speak to some people at RNLI HQ who do not know where Douglas is – or the Isle of Man, for that matter!'

Janet Kelly, Manager, Tower Lifeboat Station

Listening to Janet you can hear just how much she loves the River Thames. She says she always has done and considers herself to be a very fortunate person to have a job that brings her into such close contact with the river. She is one of three full-time RNLI employees who manage lifeboat stations on the Thames, and the only woman in this post. Janet was appointed to this responsible position in 2001 in advance of the service starting. She came with a perfect set of competencies, having spent the last five years of her thirty-year police career in the Thames Division of the Metropolitan Police.

Janet deliberately chose to work on the River Thames for the final years of her police service and had to work her way though the initial distrust she encountered from colleagues – she was the only female police sergeant on the river. Coming to the end of her commission and starting to think about what came next, she nearly missed the RNLI advertisement. Once she read the job description, she was keen to apply and subsequently very happy to be offered the post. Then, she recalls that her feet 'barely touched the ground' as she and the other managers had four months to get everything ready for the service to go live on 2 January 2002.

Janet's first-hand experience of the river was vital in helping the RNLI to shape and specify the new service. It obviously had to be operated very differently from the existing lifeboat service because the environmental, social and regulatory conditions were so differ-

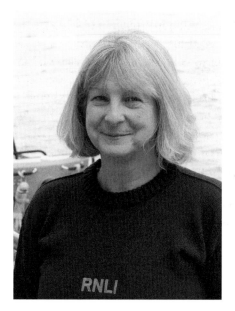

Janet Kelly, Manager of Tower Lifeboat Station.

ent from those on the coast. First and foremost, the fast tidal river water is full of dangerous and unpleasant obstacles – dead rats, excrement, needles, fat globules, shopping trolleys and trees, to name but a few. She was therefore quite certain that the lifeboat should be propelled by water jets and not by propellers.

Significant are the people issues: into London come thousands of commuters every day and millions of tourists each year, and unfortunately it attracts people who come with the intention of committing suicide. The service would be operating under the gaze of many people and not in the relative privacy out at sea. Crews would need to be trained and prepared for these conditions. They would also need to have a working knowledge of the many river byelaws. As a police officer, Janet was well aware of the security issues, which would be greater than anything the RNLI had experienced elsewhere.

It was not always easy for the RNLI to make the necessary adaptations – there were differences of understanding to be resolved. Janet remembers having big discussions about the right type of personal protection equipment for the crew. She had the confidence of specialist knowledge from her years on the river, but sometimes it was an uneasy situation for a relatively new employee. She was encouraged by the belief that the service she was helping to design was a very good thing for London. She was aware that some RNLI supporters had expressed doubts about the wisdom of establishing a lifeboat service on the River Thames, and so appreciated the consistent support she and the other managers received from then Operations Director, who expressed no doubts about the need for such a service.

For four years, Tower Lifeboat Station operated from a public pier underneath Tower Bridge in what Janet describes as a 'metal box'. It had no windows, was freezing in winter and boiling in summer and not actually in the best location for the crews to achieve the rapid response times needed. When she heard that the Metropolitan Police intended to sell Waterloo Pier, Janet knew the right person to speak to. Her enquiry met with a positive response and the happy outcome was a partnership agreement between the Metropolitan Police and the RNLI, which enabled the RNLI to purchase Waterloo Pier for just £1, and convert it into the fully functional lifeboat station that it is today.

Knowing so many key people working in many different agencies on the River Thames has definitely helped Janet in the task of developing the coordinated search and rescue service proposed by the river safety enquiry after the *Marchioness* disaster. However, it is work that requires diplomacy as well as a high level of operational competence. Eight years after the RNLI Thames lifeboat service started, Janet considers that her first invitation to the Port of London Authority annual event for all these agencies is a signal that she has made good progress!

Since its inception, the crews have been very much busier than was ever anticipated and Janet has been profoundly impressed – and amazed – by the approach of the lifeboat crews, and their commitment to doing all they can to save life in ways that are selfless, caring and non-judgemental. She has observed that even when their task is to recover a dead body, they do this respectfully with the belief that the family of the deceased should have the knowledge that everything possible had been done for their loved one. On reflection, Janet realises that she had inadvertently become accustomed to the indifference other professionals often show to death. She has been moved by the joy she sees among the lifeboat crew when they have saved a life. Somewhat to her surprise, Janet realises that working with RNLI crews has made her a more compassionate person.

After a slow start, the number of women on the crew has grown and Janet's aspiration of building teams with a good gender balance is happening. As the sole policewoman on the Thames she set out to gain respect by demonstrating her loyalty as a member of the team. Janet works hard to nurture good team skills in all the men and women on the lifeboat crews. She feels rewarded when she sees happy relationships develop and is especially pleased with the rapport that has built between the paid employees and the volunteers. Janet can see each learn from the other and the beneficial outcome of increased performance all round.

Looking forward, she would like to see more women coming forward to join lifeboat crews, not just on the River Thames but all around the coast. Janet's experience in both the police service and the RNLI has helped her to understand that many women need encouragement to recognise their abilities and often have to be helped towards achieving a level of confidence to fulfil their potential. As the manager of a lifeboat station, Janet is able to do this. Her hope is for a more collective approach from the RNLI towards active encouragement of women into volunteering for crews. Her practical experience of recruiting and developing women in her crew convinces her that there is scope for the RNLI to do some lateral thinking. As a woman who admits to exceeding her own expectations of her career, she speaks from experience.

RNLI Trustees and Council Members

Alison Saunders, the first woman Trustee

Ever since the RNLI was formed, a meeting of its Trustees was an all-male gathering. Together on stage for the annual meeting, the visual impression was that of a 'sea of suits'. That was until 2003 when the first woman Trustee, Alison Saunders, was appointed. She brought an all-important female perspective to the governance of the RNLI – and some welcome colour!

Alison's parents brought her up to believe that voluntary service should be a serious and lifelong commitment. In the early 1970s, soon after her marriage to Richard, she was therefore very responsive to the suggestion made by a friend of his that she should help the RNLI. Alison agreed, even though she had no interest in water sports, could not swim and suffered from seasickness. She has a vivid memory of the first meeting of the Central London Ladies' Committee she attended: 'A real switch off as the majority of the members were sixty plus and dressed to the nines. There was more jewellery on show than one would now wear to a City Banquet!' She declined to join.

A different experience a little later – attending the Presentation of Awards ceremony – did capture her imagination and her heart: 'As I listened to each citation, it dawned on me that here was a unique group who were prepared to risk their own lives to save individuals they didn't know and who they would probably never see again.' On the strength of this inspiration, Alison did join the Central London Ladies' Committee, where her talents were quickly recognised by the Chairman, Lady Norton. After a period as her deputy, Alison became the youngest ever Chairman of this successful committee in 1978. Lady Norton continued her support for Alison by proposing her for the RNLI Committee of Management. Alison was accepted on to the Fundraising Committee, and subsequently in 1994 she took over as Chairman. Undertaking this role meant that Alison was now also a Trustee – the first woman ever to hold that position, achieved 170 years after the RNLI was founded.

As a Trustee of a major national charity, Alison now had significant responsibilities, as well as engagements that took her all over the country. She always relished meeting the volunteers, both at lifeboat stations and among the inland fundraising branches. They enjoyed meeting her, too, as Alison has a special gift of communicating encouragement and appreciation. She also knows how to have fun, and her years in the RNLI have brought her many amusing experiences.

Perhaps it is only looking back that she can see the amusing side of her first ever lifeboat naming ceremony at Crimdon Dene on the north-east coast. It is customary to dress smartly for these occasions, but Alison did not know that she would have to struggle through high wind and driving rain across a beach to reach the ceremony site. Bedraggled best describes how she felt that day. Then she was not told that there would be 5,000 people in the audience at the Albert Hall when she went to accept a cheque from the Keep Fit Association in 1988. Alison remembers her knees knocking in fear!

Alison became Deputy Chairman of the RNLI in 2004 and retired in 2009 after thirty-six years' service. She answers with great clarity the question about what her voluntary service in the RNLI has meant to her:

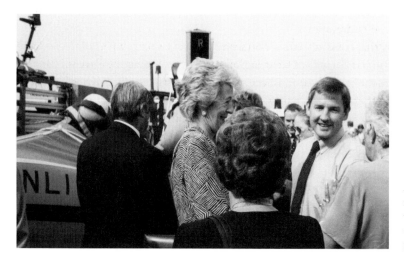

Alison Saunders mixing with RNLI volunteers at Cardigan Lifeboat Station in 1999.

Firstly, it has been a life enhancing experience, one that has brought me the opportunity to work alongside men functioning at the top of their profession. Men who never made me feel like a 'mere woman', as I suspect could have happened. Secondly, it has been a humbling experience to meet all those gallant men and women who are the face of the RNLI and who risk all with extreme modesty, total dedication and utmost efficiency.

Belinda Bucknall QC

Belinda Bucknall has been in practice as a barrister since 1975, specialising in shipping and maritime law. She joined the RNLI Council in 2007.

Born in Wargrave in Berkshire, which Belinda describes as 'just about as far from the sea as it is possible to be in England', she recalls a childhood affinity with the water and was then an enthusiastic raft builder on the River Thames. It was probably this, she thinks, that triggered her lifelong passion for water transport, from which she has built her career.

Her initial contact with the RNLI came at about the age of six when her school held a fête in aid of the lifeboat service. Belinda made and sold a large number of buttonholes, mainly using pansies and dandelions. Even the dead ones sold, which, she suggests, shows just how willing people are to support their favourite charity!

Belinda has acted for the RNLI in a number of cases, including the Public Inquiry into the loss of the Penlee lifeboat. It was during the course of those proceedings that she recalls:

> I really came to understand what sacrifices my fellow countrymen, including their families, make to save lives at sea. I have been involved in numbers of cases involving shipping disasters in UK waters, where the RNLI lifeboat crews have performed feats of true heroism in rescuing the crews of stricken vessels, in the case of yachts and small commercial vessels, quite often saving the vessels as well.

Being associated with the RNLI and being able to make a professional contribution behind the scenes does therefore mean a great deal to Belinda. She is impressed by the professional way in which the organisation is run and how much care is taken to ensure donations are spent in the best possible way to further the charitable purposes. What she particularly likes is the way the RNLI draws people together from every part of the country, both from coastal and from inland communities.

Belinda's love of rafting has never left her, and every year she spends a part of the summer rafting or canoeing in the far north of Canada. Somewhere in that distant place is an RNLI fleece, which a Canadian First Nations fisheries officer was thrilled to receive as a gift after towing Belinda and her raft for several miles when strong headwinds stopped her dead in the water! 'Hopefully he is still wearing it because the thought does so please me that all those miles away on the other side of the North Atlantic the logo is being displayed by someone who so clearly supports the values of the RNLI.'

Ann Watkin

Ann Watkin is now retired, but has had a successful career in retailing and consumer affairs. Additionally, she has served on a number of public bodies, notably as Director of the Scottish Consumer Council, and Chairman of the Consumer Panel of the Financial

Services Authority. She joined the RNLI Council in 2002 and has been a member of the Fundraising and Communications Committee since 2001.

Ann had no connection with the sea at all and so had no preconceptions about the RNLI when she was first approached to become involved. She recalls her early impressions of the organisation as rather 'stuffy', traditional and very much male dominated. She felt that it was run rather too much along service lines, being very formal and highly control-led. For her, there was a real question: 'I did not think I could make much of a contribution to what looked very much like an old boys' club.'

The motivation to stay was partly provided by Alison Saunders, who was then Chairman of the Fundraising and Communications Committee: 'I have the highest regard for Alison – far better than most of the chaps put together!' Her growing understanding of the complex and sophisticated fundraising function within the organisation was also a contributory factor. Introduction to the work of the volunteer fundraisers encouraged Ann to get involved herself, and she now chairs the Harrogate Ladies' Lifeboat Guild. Here she sees first-hand the 'amazing commitment' of the volunteers – mostly women – and how hard they work to raise funds.

Reflecting upon the title of this book, Ann suspects that 'most of the RNLI women are unsung heroes – the kind of people who work hard in a modest way and who care little about rank or titles'. She has, however, seen change during the decade of her involvement and, with more women in senior positions, believes that the organisation is the better for it. Her hope is that the number of women in senior positions will continue to increase.

Rosie Allen-Mirehouse

Rosie Allen-Mirehouse has held a number of varied roles. Firstly, she has worked for *The Sunday Telegraph* as secretary to the Literary Editor; she has also cooked at a couple of hotels in West Wales and spent a year at Highgrove as Cook/Housekeeper to the Prince and Princess of Wales. She joined the RNLI Council in 2008.

It was her experience of meeting members of the crew and volunteers in St David's that was Rosie's first real encounter with the RNLI. If that could be described as dipping her toes in the water, then marriage to John Allen-Mirehouse was total immersion! For a start, John is the long serving Lifeboat Operations Manager of Angle Lifeboat Station, but as Rosie explains: 'When a remote village like Angle has a lifeboat, it is impossible *not* to be involved. The whole community is connected somehow – lifeboat families go back four or five generations and many of the Angle families are related and interconnected in some way.'

Rosie is 'immersed' in several ways. She is a Deputy Launching Authority at the station, meaning that she is one of just three people at Angle Lifeboat Station who is authorised to make the judgement whether to launch the lifeboat when a request is received. It is therefore a very responsible role requiring sound nautical knowledge, and Rosie has vivid memories of the first launch she authorised – her thoughts were with the crew families at home throughout the rescue. She is a member of the Angle Fundraising Committee and President of Pembroke Ladies' Lifeboat Guild.

The RNLI has become a very important part of Rosie's life and she is quite clear about the source of her motivation: 'I just need to see our lifeboat go down the slipway in foul, dark weather.' Appealing to Rosie is the determination of the organisation to maintain its financial independence, together with its strong volunteer ethic. It is her first-hand experience of volunteers and her understanding of the operation of the lifeboat service that Rosie brings to the deliberations of the Council.

She is clearly a strong advocate for all those who volunteer, seeking only to support the work of the crews:

> I want to mention the many unnamed, faithful fundraisers who stand in the rain and cold outside supermarkets, train stations and street corners with collecting boxes and buckets. It is a thankless task and not one of the RNLI's biggest fundraising profiles, but to me they are the public front of RNLI fundraising, and no-one will ever know how many people see such dedication and so decide to make a will in favour of the RNLI.

Dame Valerie Strachan DBE

Dame Valerie Strachan retired ten years ago from her role as Chairman of the Board of HM Customs. Now she is involved with a variety of activities including the Big Lottery Fund. She is Chair of the Council of Southampton University and Chair of James Allen's Girls' School. She joined the RNLI Council in 1993.

Dame Valerie first became involved through the Civil Service Lifeboat Fund, which has a long history of raising money for the RNLI. She explains that there was a natural connection between the RNLI and Customs because the revenue cutters and relations between the two organisations have always been good. The Civil Service Lifeboat Fund is actually the longest standing supporter of the RNLI. It made the first donation for a lifeboat in 1866 and since then has donated sufficient to fund a further forty-three lifeboats, the most recent being *Public Servant (Civil Service No. 44)* stationed on the River Thames.

Her early impression of the RNLI was of 'wonderful people' working in a slightly old-fashioned organisation. Over the years of her involvement Dame Valerie has seen it develop hugely into a modern forward-looking outfit – but still full of wonderful people. For her, this is a good reason why she and her Civil Service colleagues should continue to give their support.

RNLI staff

Paid staff are far fewer in number than volunteers, but there has been a parallel increase in the number of employees as the organisation has expanded and diversified. The first women employees worked in traditional office roles at the London-based headquarters, but all other posts were held by men. The mould was at last broken when, in post-war years, women were appointed to the role of District Organising Secretary. The purpose of this job was to provide professional support to the volunteer fundraising committees. These women opened the door, and since then many others have walked through to undertake a wide range of responsibilities.

In 2010, the RNLI employs 489 women – approximately 40 per cent of the workforce. These are just some of them, predominantly those who have been 'firsts' or who have broken new ground for the RNLI.

Ali Peck, HR and Training Director, First Woman Executive Board Member

One year after the first female Trustee was appointed, a woman was appointed to the Executive Board – just one month after the 180th anniversary of the founding of the RNLI. Even though this seems to have been slow in coming, by comparison with other major UK employers, the organisation had done quite well. In 2010, just 10 per cent of board members of FTSE 100 companies are women.

In 1999, having pursued her career as a manager in the private and public sectors, Ali had decided to make a move into the human resources profession. It was a coincidence, she reflects, that the RNLI was recruiting HR advisers at the same time, and pure chance that she saw the advertisement. Her parents had both had longstanding involvement with the RNLI – her father through maritime interests and her mother on the fundraising side, so Ali was familiar with the charity. When she started work at HQ in Poole, she experienced an instant affinity – it was a place where people mattered and values were important, where she felt the sense of family, and yet everything the RNLI did was highly professional. She knew it all felt right for her.

Five years later she was offered a position on the Executive Board as Human Resources Director and she accepted. Ali says that many people have asked her what it feels like to be the only woman in this team. She readily acknowledges that it has not always been easy; a group that has always comprised men only has very distinctive and established ways of operating – not always easy for women to fit into and not one that can change overnight to assimilate female values and preferences. However, Ali confirms that she has come to greatly enjoy and value the working relationships with her male colleagues on the board and she believes that, as a women, her presence is helpful in eliciting different behaviours in group situations. She is convinced that she has always had the sense of being an equal player and has never felt patronised. Most importantly, her areas of responsibility, now HR and Training, have been given the level of strategic importance they should have.

Her answer is a definite 'yes' to the question 'Would it be good to have more women on the board and in senior management posts?', but Ali thinks there are a number of reasons why this might not be easy to achieve. She sees that there are certainly many women who have not had the opportunities to develop themselves and their career, and accepting this, she is keen that the RNLI as an employer should be more aware of how it can support women in a positive way. Perhaps a more significant reason, though, is that many women choose not to put themselves forward for the most senior positions. Ali attributes this to innate differences between male and female motivations; women tend to recognise the 'politicking and game playing' often associated with senior status and find those behaviours difficult and stressful. They are far less interested in overt forms of recognition and much more motivated to achieve something worthwhile, which experience tells them is more likely to be possible in roles of lesser status.

When Ali looks at the employment statistics for the RNLI – which show that while 47 per cent of the workforce is female, just 22 per cent of those women are senior managers – she is concerned that the percentage should improve, but takes heart that she has seen movement in the right direction. She knows that if her interpretations of why women do not present themselves for more senior posts are correct, there are some barriers to

Ali Peck, HR and Training Director, inside the Lifeboat College in 2008.

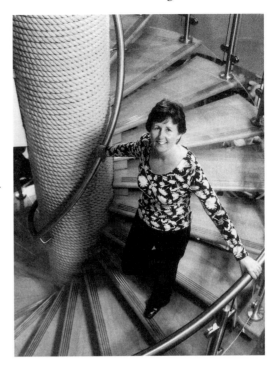

remove so that the organisational culture becomes more conducive to women. Ali wants to see more women in key positions, but she is convinced that they have to be appointed for the right reasons; for the skills and knowledge they can bring to work for the benefit of the RNLI. 'Balanced teams are the best teams,' says Ali. 'Men and women have different skills and the best outcomes are to be had when a team draws upon the full complement of what both men and women can offer'.

Ali considers this to be as true within the volunteer community of the RNLI as the paid staff. Just 10 per cent of lifeboat crew members are women and 27 per cent of lifeboat stations have no women crew at all. The proportion in lifeguarding is higher; 20 per cent of lifeguards are women. Her aspiration is for more women to feel motivated to present themselves as operational volunteers and, just as importantly, feel welcomed and valued and so want to stay.

Describing the women of the RNLI as 'just extraordinary', Ali has observed many different women in every part of the organisation. She has seen them to be hugely engaged and passionate about whatever it is they do to help save lives at sea. Sometimes this involves them having to be very resilient and tenacious, breaking through long-established barriers. She has perceived their 'hidden depths': 'Working behind the scenes … just getting on with it, without the need for praise or recognition; quietly bringing order to disorder; making peace; smoothing things out'. As her list builds, Ali pauses and reflects: 'It poses a question; where would the RNLI be without them?'

Sarah Nimmo-Scott, first Deputy Divisional Inspector of Lifeboats

Lifeboat Inspectors fulfil an important role in the RNLI. They have front line responsibility on the coast for the overall management of lifeboat crews, volunteer and employed staff, the station premises, lifeboats and other equipment, as well as training and assessment. They must ensure compliance with all relevant safety standards and legislation. Through them the high operational standards for which the RNLI is renowned are upheld. Candidates for the position will only be recruited if they have significant and credible maritime experience and are able to demonstrate well-honed interpersonal skills. The selection bar is set high and until very recently only men have crossed it. Sarah Nimmo-Scott is the first woman in this post, and while she is not intimidated by this distinction, she does take her job very seriously.

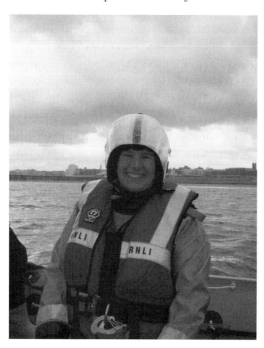

Sarah Nimmo-Scott, Deputy Divisional Inspector of Lifeboats.

This is not the first time she has been the only female in a male dominated environment. On leaving her all-girls school she studied Mechanical Engineering at Bristol University. She then joined the Royal Navy and served for five years at sea on various ships. Subsequent employment included training fishermen in sea survival and project management in an electrical engineering company. Sarah taught navigation and seamanship in the Royal Naval Reserve. It is therefore hardly surprising that she has robust convictions about female competency:

> During all these roles the one thing that struck me was not so much whether I was a woman or not but how well I could do my job and get on with people. I think this is true for all walks of life and as a result I have never felt marginalized or discriminated against by virtue of being a woman.

A woman Lifeboat Inspector was such a significant departure within the organisation that, inevitably, some voices questioned how she would be received on the coast, given that most lifeboat crew are male. Again, Sarah responded very pragmatically:

> I think maybe they underestimated our lifeboat crews most of whom live in the outside world where women have been doing the same jobs as men for a very long time. Lifeboating has traditionally been a male preserve but as long as we have the most capable people going to sea on our lifeboats then we are doing the right thing.

Sarah works in the RNLI North Division, which stretches along the west coast from the Solway Firth to the Mersey Estuary, and along the east coast from Berwick-upon-Tweed to the Wash. With thirty-three lifeboat stations, it is no wonder she has such a busy and varied life. The best bits so far? Delivering new inshore lifeboats to stations and training the crews on the differences with the new boat, is the answer: 'They are all really proud of their old boats and have confidence in them, having used them for so many shouts in the past. When you bring them a new boat it is the start of a new relationship for them.'

Anne Millman, first Youth Promotion Coordinator

A major challenge for a charity that relies on voluntary income is to ensure that the next generation has an awareness of and willingness to engage with the cause. It was for just this purpose that the post of Youth Promotion Coordinator (now the National Education Manager) was created in 1993, and it was Anne Millman, a science teacher on the Isle of Wight, who was the successful applicant. Anne was a keen sailor and had already experienced the work of the RNLI in 1992 through an Industry/Education Exchange placement at the Inshore Lifeboat Centre at Cowes.

What a huge task faced her when she started work at HQ in November 1993. There was precious little RNLI precedent for a strategic approach to engaging young people and so, faced with a blank sheet of paper, she identified two lines of approach: to produce resources for schools and to develop a network of education officers who would be able to engage relationships with schools and youth organisations within each RNLI region.

As a teacher, Anne knew there was a great opportunity to link any new resources with the national curriculum. In fact, this would probably be the only way of attracting the attention of schools, which would struggle to take on anything else in these early days of the national curriculum. The first focus was on seven to eleven year olds, with a resource pack called *Launch!*, which included a lively video. Take up from schools was good, and the pack received a commendation from the *Times Educational Supplement*.

Sometimes it is difficult to get confirmation that educational messages are having an impact, but Anne recalls that when Youth Education linked up with the RNLI Sea Safety team to produce *Get Splashed* – a guide for children and families on how to keep safe in and around the water – there was great feedback from schools, youth organisations, local authorities and lifeboat stations that attitudes to safety were improving. It was also motivating to discover that there was a marked uptake of RNLI material in school textbooks and that the Qualifications and Curriculum Authority had selected RNLI material for the English SATs tests – translating it into Braille too.

Following a competition in *Storm Force News*, the magazine for the RNLI's children's membership, and then in conjunction with Georgette Purches, Deputy Head of Public Relations, Stormy Stan burst upon the world at around this time and soon gathered a strong following in the magazine as well as becoming the figure that the children wanted to see at fundraising events. Anne remembers herself wearing the Stormy Stan suit around the HQ and, well hidden as she was, having fun at the expense of a senior manager who, without success, tried to insist on knowing who was inside.

With the clear success of the resources strategy, the RNLI took the decision to pilot in three regions Anne's proposal for a network of education officers. It worked well and now there are officers in each region, each making great strides to engage younger people to know about and have a willingness to support the RNLI. A Child Protection Policy was developed in tandem with further resources for young people, for teachers of five to fourteen year olds, and for volunteers and fundraisers working with children. Anne, who now works as a freelance consultant, is happy that a lot has been achieved since 1993, but notes that other major charities are very active in engaging youth, and she believes that the RNLI would be wise to do even more to attract future generations.

Anne is one of the women of the RNLI who is both an employee and a volunteer crew member. She already had some experience of crewing on the then independent Cowes Inshore Rescue boat (which became an RNLI lifeboat station in 2008), but when she was settled in Poole she decided to volunteer for the Poole lifeboat. On speaking to her manager of this intention, she was dismayed by a somewhat lukewarm response and later learned he was concerned that, with Poole being such a busy lifeboat station, Anne might be forever rushing away from her work on a shout. The matter was resolved up the line by Ray Kipling, Deputy Director, who said: 'Well, if we can't let her go, how can we expect other employers to release staff?'

There was a second hurdle – at the lifeboat station. Poole already had two women crew members and the reaction Anne experienced from the men was the question: 'How many more females do we want?' There were also concerns that, as she worked at HQ, how were they to know 'how she wore her hat' when in her crew role at the station? Anne was philosophical about this, knowing that her loyalty to the crew would be absolute.

After many months of training she was accepted as a full crew member. Poole is one of the busiest stations on the coast, and so, after fifteen years on the crew, she has undertaken many rescues. The one that really stands out for her is when she helped rescue a man who had become trapped against the side of the Chain Ferry at the mouth of Poole Harbour – his wife had already gone under the ferry and had been rescued by the crew on the Brede class lifeboat:

> As I hung over the side of the inshore lifeboat clutching hold of his hand with all my strength, in spite of all that was going on around me, I suddenly had the thought – I *literally* have this man's life in my hand. It was profound.

Anne often cites Ellen MacArthur when questions are asked about how women can cope with the physical rigours of lifeboating. She points out that Ellen is small in stature and yet achieves great things through her skill and determination. Anne needed both those in the Chain Ferry rescue and was very happy afterwards to receive a Framed Letter of Thanks from the RNLI's Chairman: 'I knew what a difficult rescue it was but it was good to know that someone else had also recognised it.'

There was a 'work-versus-crew' occasion when Anne was in full flow giving a presentation to the Director and Senior Managers at a crowded meeting in the HQ building. Suddenly her pager went off. Anne's hand automatically went to her belt to turn off the pager, but then she looked aghast and turned to Brian Miles, the Director, and said: 'Can I go?' With a beaming smile, he said: 'I think you better had!' Anne fled, leaving everyone in the room roaring with laughter.

Having a good – some might call it 'black' – sense of humour is essential on a lifeboat crew, whether you are a man or a woman. Anne has a catalogue of funny stories, which includes one about a night when red flares were sighted in Poole Harbour, but, try as they might, the crew just could not find where they were coming from. After some time, they heard gunshots coming from one of the small islands in the harbour. As they edged gently closer, all suddenly became clear – there were people shooting rabbits on the island and they were wearing infrared headband torches. When the smoke from the gun drifted into

Anne Millman, formerly Youth Promotion Coordinator and member of Poole lifeboat crew.

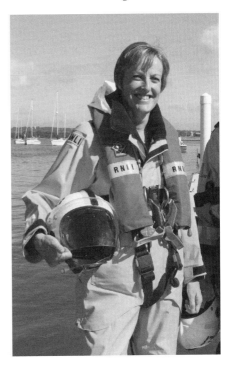

the torchlight it looked just like a red flare! The local press were also attracted by the story:

Hundreds of Lives Saved ... probably

When Poole's Atlantic launched at 20.50 on Easter Saturday this year [1999] the crew thought they were searching for red flares. Instead, when they arrived at the scene in a dark and uninhabited corner of Poole Harbour, they found moving infrared lights – and the sound of shotguns!

A substantial number of Easter Bunnies were seen diving for cover, and the lifeboat crew – very wisely – decided not to go ashore just yet!

The arrival of a rather official looking boat with a blue light – even if it was a little reluctant to come too close – evidently distracted the marksmen, and as their lights faded rapidly away the rabbit population headed for its burrows.

Crewmember Anne Millman later attributed the Cause of Service to 'Rabbits in Distress'; the Prime Cause of Incident as 'Shotgun Held at Nose Point' and the Total Number of Survivors as 'lots', adding that there would have been hundreds more by the end of the shout …

Anne works at the Poole HQ spearheading the RNLI's youth promotion campaign and producing *Storm Force News*, so perhaps it's just as well that her younger readers won't hear her final remark: The crew won't be claiming salvage, but some rabbit pie wouldn't have gone amiss. Happy Easter!

Holly Phillips, first woman RNLI Principle Naval Architect

Growing up in Wimbledon seems an unlikely background for a girl who loved the sea and boats so much that she was determined to become a naval architect and, if at all possible, work for the RNLI. The explanation is that Holly had a grandfather who owned a house in Swanage and so she and her family spent most summer holidays there.

'The house was close to the lifeboat station so I got into the lifeboating zone from an early age,' explains Holly. She would rush down to see the launch when the maroons went off and so got to know the crew quite well. In her teenage years she worked for Marsh's Pleasure Boats on Swanage Quay and took every opportunity to build up her skills and increase her knowledge of boats and the sea in readiness for her naval architecture studies.

Holly secured a degree place at Southampton University and found she was the only girl in her year. She is very clear that she was not daunted by having twenty-nine male peers: 'I just wanted to be good at what I did', but she believes this student experience, combined with that of working on the boats in Swanage and the friendships she had made there, gave her a natural style in working with men. This was to be of great benefit to her in both her career path and in her decision to volunteer as a lifeboat crew member.

In an endeavour to get a foot in the door of the RNLI as her employer of choice and to do work that would have a tangible benefit, Holly skilfully used the project element of her degree. She sent a proposal to the RNLI Engineering Office to look at possible differences in strength between composites with stitched fabrics as compared with those using woven. The RNLI was at that time designing two new classes of lifeboat (the FAB3 and FAB4, later to become the Severn and Trent), so the proposal was timely and Holly's project was accepted. It was a good experience for Holly and confirmed for her that the RNLI was where she eventually wanted to work.

In 1994 she just happened to be in the right place at the right time when the coxswain of Poole lifeboat, finding he was short of crew for a shout, asked her if she would join them to look for a lost windsurfer. Holly jumped at the opportunity and the experience was such that soon afterwards she wrote to the Honorary Secretary asking if she could join the Poole lifeboat crew. After a six-month probation period and the crew vote, she was accepted and made history by being both the first female crew member at Poole Lifeboat Station, and the 100th female crew member in the RNLI as a whole.

She recalls that her reception from Poole crew was very positive and encouraging. Holly believes that this is partly due to the experience of boating she brought and the fact that she was a willing learner. Her chance status as the 100th woman crew member brought unexpected publicity, which drew comments from some of the other crew, but Holly remembers that the majority of those at the station were very supportive and soon the spotlight on Holly faded and she was able to focus on her training and gaining invaluable experience as a crew member.

Holly has now served on the crew for sixteen years and is now a helm on Poole's inshore lifeboat. She readily acknowledges that a lot has changed in this time in terms of the boats, crew and society generally. She is quick to recognise how much more thorough the training is now, but reflects that there is still a place for local training and that it would be a real loss to RNLI crews if this were to be ignored. Perhaps influenced by the fact that Poole is such a busy lifeboat station in a tourist locality, she is conscious of how the lifeboat service seems to be increasingly taken for granted by the public who use it as a free 'get home' service and by those (albeit a minority) who manipulate the system to get a free tow in. On balance, though, she believes firmly in the value of what the lifeboat crew does and says how good it is to receive the thanks of the people genuinely in trouble.

Recalling the memorable shouts, she tells the story of one that left her absolutely exhausted. It was to a boat that had become stranded on the mud in Poole Harbour: 'We had to get to it by walking across the mud dragging an X Boat to bring the people back in. It was so difficult – I felt almost dead at the end! I knew, though, that if it wasn't for us, those people would have been in real trouble'. On a memorable August bank holiday weekend in 1995, Poole's lifeboats (there were four on station that weekend) carried out thirty-two services. Holly was in the thick of it all and remembers how tiring but exhilarating it was, spending virtually the entire weekend rescuing people in trouble.

In 2001, after having spent several years designing ship's rudders, she spotted a job advert and applied for a position in the RNLI's Technical Department in Poole. Her application

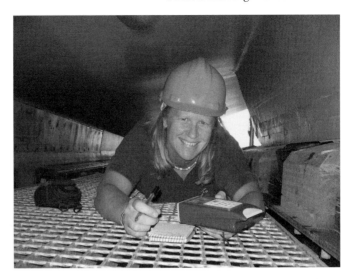

Holly Phillips, Senior Naval
Architect and member of
Poole lifeboat crew.

was successful and Holly started work there in 2002. With both childhood ambitions fulfilled and doing something that she truly enjoys, Holly went from strength to strength and
is now the RNLI's Principal Naval Architect. She uses her sharp knowledge of lifeboating
in her professional role: 'There are huge benefits – when I am designing a new piece of kit,
I already have a good understanding of what will work and so the process is more stream-
lined'.

Her pride in the RNLI is tangible, as is her desire for the strengths of the organisation to
be used even more effectively in the cause of saving lives at sea:

> I understand that new ideas can take a long time to work through but I firmly believe that we
> have the opportunity to use technology and resources in the right way and so further improve
> the RNLI service. That's what I want to help make happen in the future!

Helena Duggan, first woman Divisional Assessor Trainer

Helena works for the RNLI as a Divisional Assessor Trainer – she is the first woman to
be appointed to this post, and as yet, she is the only woman in the team, which covers the
UK and the Republic of Ireland, where she is based. Her work requires her to have high
levels of experience and personal competence in the knowledge and skills that the RNLI
considers essential for lifeboat crew to possess. In 2002, when Competence Based Training
was introduced in the RNLI, there was a need to employ qualified assessors (later training
was added to their remit) around the coast to make objective assessments to validate the
required levels of competency achieved by each man and woman serving on a RNLI crew.

The position interested Helena who, living in County Wexford, had volunteered for
Courtown lifeboat crew in 1989. She was keen on water sports and was a beach lifeguard
with Irish Water Safety, so joining the lifeboat crew of a station which was just about to
be reopened after almost 100 years was very appealing. It was a very positive experience,
which confirmed for Helena that women can make an equal contribution when saving
lives at sea. She takes immense pride both in the RNLI and the service it provides and what

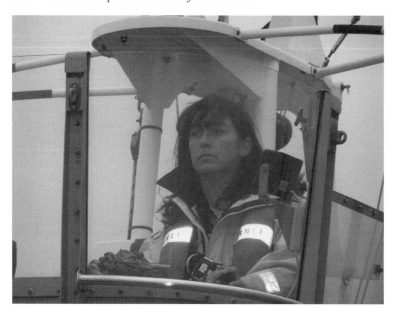

Helena Duggan, Divisional Assessor Trainer and member of Courtown lifeboat crew.

she is able to offer: 'I don't look upon it as something out of the ordinary or it affecting my life … it just *is* my life'. She is now one of the helms of Courtown lifeboat.

As an experienced volunteer crew member, Helena had just the right background to achieve credibility as an ambassador of the new Competence Based Training. She would like to think that she is accepted at lifeboat stations for the level of work and commitment she gives in her role and would prefer it if the fact that she is a woman is not noticed in the context of what she contributes to the advancement and growth of the RNLI. Helena quite clearly rejects positive discrimination towards women in recruiting lifeboat crews:

> I don't think women should be on lifeboats to address 'gender balance', but that every person should be treated as an individual, regardless of sex. People who are prepared to volunteer their time and risk their lives for others should be respected for their strength and helped with their weaknesses. We depend on each other for so much at sea.

Helena is simply amused by the surprise of some people when they find they have been rescued by a woman crewing an inshore lifeboat. Now that she is qualified to coxswain level and has authority to take all-weather lifeboats on passage, there may be more surprises to come …

Jill Hepburn, first woman Senior Trainer

Jill's father had a favourite saying: 'He who hesitates is lost'. When a vacancy for an inshore lifeboat trainer came up in 2005, she remembered his words, took the plunge, and applied. After what she describes as a tough interview, she got the job. Jill's motivation to train lifeboat crew came from the very positive experience she herself had of an RNLI training course when she was a member of Ballyglass lifeboat crew. Of course when she moved to work in the Lifeboat College at Poole she had, with regret, to leave the crew.

From Ballyglass she brought valuable lifeboating experience, but she believes she has been fortunate on more than one account:

> Firstly, I've been raised to believe that I can do the same things as men can do, but like anyone have limitations which I recognise. Secondly, ever since joining Ballyglass crew I was just one of the team who gave as good as I got and just got on with it. If you lead by example, get stuck in and don't make an issue of being the only woman, then it isn't one.

This is the philosophy she brings to work in the RNLI Training Department, and her promotion to Senior Trainer – the first woman ever to hold this position – reinforced her conviction that if you lead by example, you get the support of your team which, at present, is all male. Jill acknowledges that probably she cramps their style on 'boys' nights', but has been told that she is the 'token lad'. Although not sure what that means, she recognises it as a backhanded compliment. She does sometimes see herself as a calming influence in the team.

Jill loves her job, believing that she is an exception to the view that you should never make your hobby your job. She feels rewarded when letters of appreciation and thanks come from crew who have enjoyed and valued the training. Her family are proud and supportive of what she does as they do a lot of sailing and understand the value of the RNLI. Like Jill, they know how important it is for the volunteer crew to be trained well so that they can operate safely when saving the lives of others. Jill is convinced that her time as a crew member has helped her be an effective trainer. She has first-hand experience of mutual reliance and the need for teamwork with everyone looking out for each other – so great is the sense of family.

Out in Poole Bay is Jill's workplace – in the sunshine (sometimes!), on a lifeboat with a crew in training. No wonder her granny called her 'my Action Girl'.

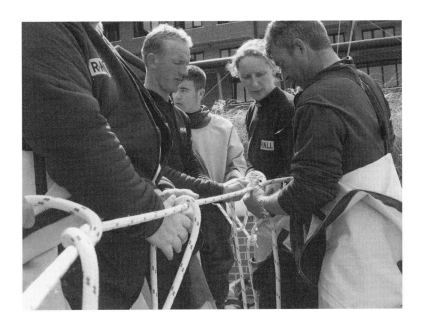

Jill Hepburn
teaching knots
at the Lifeboat
College, Poole.

Val Nixon, Senior Fundraising Manager, and woman with longest RNLI employment service

Val is just a few months away from her retirement date and has more than just a strange feeling about what that will be like. She has worked for the RNLI since 1967 when she was a sixteen-year-old school leaver. After forty-four years, her life and the RNLI have become woven so closely together that separating them seems unreal. Val is the longest serving woman employee, which is something of a miracle as she intended only to stay for three months until the job she really wanted became available! Her teenage dream was of working in a smart high-rise office block in York and Yorkshire General Insurance offered her one, but there was a snag. The job would not be available for another three months. 'Not likely!' said her mother. 'Go and get something now.'

So she did: a temporary clerical post with the RNLI, in a very non-smart low-rise office in York. It would fill the gap. There was to be no gap, though, as Val loved the work and the people immediately: 'They were warm and friendly and keen to help me. I sensed that if I couldn't cope, others could – and would. It was a real family feeling,' remembers Val. Fortunately she had taken typing lessons at night school which gave her a valuable skill, and at the end of three months she was asked if she would be interested to take a permanent post as secretary. She thought about it … but only for about five minutes! Much to her amazement her wages rose from £5 per week to £5 10s.

The delight of the job was in helping the volunteers with whatever they were doing for the RNLI. Sometimes it was providing them with information they needed, but she also produced fundraising materials for them such as tickets, programmes and posters. All the office processes were manual; committee records were on index cards, copies were made on carbon paper, tickets were printed on a gestetner duplicator – 'and what a mess that made of our hands', she recalls. There was a great camaraderie between the staff and the volunteers, who would call into the office and telephone to organise their requests. 'A big event was when a coxswain telephoned – that was exciting'. Val took great pride in making sure that everything was just right so that her boss, Ken Thirlwell, could do his job well. That was the office ethic of the time, but additionally she had a huge personal respect for him.

A surprising opportunity came her way when she was eighteen. She was asked to work at RNLI HQ in Grosvenor Gardens, in London, for a fortnight to collect information for an alderman who was researching the history of lifeboats donated by the City of Bradford. Val had never been to London in her life but agreed to do it and spent the two weeks manually copying information from old ledgers into notes to bring back to Yorkshire. Which hotel had she stayed in? 'Hotel! You're joking … I had to stay with one of the girls from the typing pool'. Clearly she did well, because she was running the whole office by the time she was twenty.

The office was relocated to Pateley Bridge in 1975 where Val helped with setting up the new lifeboat supplies depot which shared the site. Marriage to John Parker in 1983 brought new happiness, but one that was not to last because he very sadly died five years later. For Val, who had been office-based for twenty-one years, it was time to make a move. She would dearly have liked to apply for the post of Area Organiser for North Yorkshire. It would take her out and about working directly with the volunteers, but she did not drive. She was encouraged to apply and was then offered the job on the proviso that she had passed her driving test by 1 March 1988. That mission was accomplished on 29 February! There have been some boundary changes and alterations of job title, but essentially Val has been working in this role ever since, and has relished all the challenges and achievements – but very especially, the people. People who have become firm friends.

She recalls the highlights as the events she was involved with for the RNLI's 175th anniversary in 1999, especially the magnificent service of thanksgiving in York Minster and the Gala at York Race Course, not to forget the Lifeboat Pull from Whitby to Robin Hood's Bay – a hugely successful event but one which, as Val puts it, 'turned my hair grey'. They have given her memories that she treasures. In that very busy year she had a happy personal event when she married Kevin Nixon.

But then, over forty-four years, there are so many memories to treasure. One very different one was in December 1981, when the crew of the Penlee lifeboat were all drowned. There was so much snow and ice on the roads around Pateley Bridge on Friday 18 December that they closed the office and depot early so that people could get home. During the weekend, Val learned of what had happened in Cornwall and knew she had somehow to get back into the office the following morning. Both she and Terry Burden, manager of the depot, arrived to ringing telephones – people who wanted to donate to the Penlee disaster fund. Between them they answered the calls, giving the necessary information about how to donate. Then with great difficulty because of sheet ice and snow drifts, they managed to load a van with lifeboat collecting boxes, which Terry subsequently delivered to strategic points so that volunteers could use them while the public were anxious to give.

For a person who remembers with horror the arrival of electronic typewriters in the office, Val considers that the most significant changes she has experienced in her

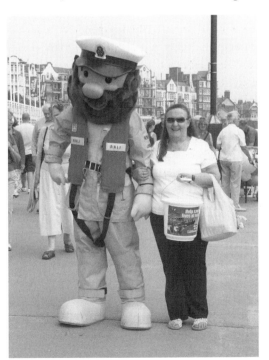

forty-four years have been technology related. Certainly there have been many of these in the office environment and she readily sees how beneficial they have been in supporting volunteers. On the coast she has seen advances in technology that have brought faster, safer lifeboats, better launching equipment, and personal protection kit for the crews. All these are very positive and welcome. As is her observation that senior people are now more approachable than when she started work. For her, this has to be a better way of running the service, which draws on the generosity and skills of people from many different backgrounds.

Val Nixon, Senior Fundraising Manager/ North.

Val has no doubt that it is the people who matter. Throughout her career, she has witnessed the motivation of people who want to support the bravery of lifeboat crews, and says that in essence this has never changed. Just as they know the crews will do, people want to go the extra mile to help: 'Both on the coast and inland there is a special camaraderie and friendship that come with belonging to the lifeboat family'.

The Rubber Solutionists, RNLI Inshore Lifeboat Centre

It is not hard to imagine the sorts of comments that come back when you give the answer 'Rubber Solutionist' when asked 'what's your job?' The team at the Inshore Lifeboat Centre at East Cowes, Isle of Wight have heard them all. Most often they are known as 'Solutionists', but then people think they are problem solvers. Very often, that is exactly what they do, according to Nicky Stokes, Assistant Production Manager and leader of a team of twenty-seven who contribute to the building and maintenance of RNLI inshore lifeboats at this 'factory with a difference'.

At what is now an internationally recognised centre of excellence for its work, women have been at the forefront of the very specialist work that Solutionists do. In fact, at one time it was solely women who performed all the intricate processes involved in gluing the inflatable section of the lifeboat to the hull as well as creating and fixing the wide range of fittings that have to be added to make a basic RIB into a fully functional lifeboat. This is exacting work, which requires careful planning, and high levels of precision in execution. Not everyone would have the patience to do this work, and it is found more frequently in women than in men.

Speak to any of the Solutionists and each will confirm without hesitation why this attention to detail and emphasis on high quality is essential. The quality of their work could make the difference between life and death. They know that when the lifeboat – one that is held together with glue – is out on a rescue it must not fail. The department also has an important role in the servicing and repair of lifejackets and, as probably the most important lifesaving equipment in the event of a capsize, they have to be cared for impeccably.

The pride that the Solutionists have in their work is tangible and is reflected in the fact that many have worked at this job for years. Known by the others as 'The Oracle', Julie Mogg has the longest service – thirty-four years. She can tell stories of the early days when they used household irons to heat up the materials, and when she had to crawl inside the sponson tube with a light bulb to find faults and then return with a pot of glue to mend them. Asked how that made her feel, she thinks for a while and says 'floaty' – which has to be an understatement! Jackie Wright, with twenty-eight years' service, did the same, and reflects on what the Heath and Safety people would say about that now – it would certainly not be allowed.

There have been huge advances in Health and Safety practices at the Inshore Lifeboat Centre over the years, as the RNLI will never compromise the safety of staff or volunteers. The glue is very powerful and each worker has to be regularly monitored for any adverse effects. Natasha Cook, who is expecting her first baby, has to wear a monitor during her working hours and feels confident that her best interests are being cared for. Much of the risk is reduced by a sophisticated air-filtering system.

Most of the women got to know about the job by word of mouth, as so often happens in a small community like East Cowes. What they discovered when they joined took many of them by surprise, having had no idea that inshore lifeboats were held together by glue nor how complex was the work required to make this happen. For those who shared the RNLI's insistence on 'second to none' quality, it was the perfect job. For Elaine Cole, who started sixteen years ago, there was an instant match. She had always supported the RNLI and was not at all disappointed with what she found as an employee: 'The high standard required fitted perfectly with me and I still love the work after all these years'. Deanne Coxhead, with a similar length of service, loves the work too, relishing all the technical challenges and the opportunity to make a contribution to new developments. She has been involved with several projects developing different fittings for radio and flare stowage, as well as creating seats for the Atlantic 85 lifeboat.

Theresa Pragnell works on some of the more intricate fittings and points out how easy it is to overlook what has gone into making something like a stowage bag. However, to be sure that they are watertight and really user friendly in the sea conditions the crews will meet, a lot of precise measuring, cutting and stitching must be done. This is confirmed by her colleague, Vicki Cotton, who is a newcomer to the Inshore Lifeboat Centre, but because she is a volunteer on The Ryde Inshore Rescue, an independent service, she understands fully the need for supplying crews with high quality kit. Admitting to having had her eyes opened by how things are done at the Inshore Lifeboat Centre, and recognising how easy it is to take so much for granted, she is very happy with her new job: 'If you've put your name on it, you want to be proud of it.'

Section Leader Patti Urry, with thirty-two years' service, is happy that she can pass on her skills and knowledge not only to her team, but also directly to the crews through training sessions at the Inshore Lifeboat Centre. The aim is to teach them gluing procedures so they know how to do small repairs at station. Some of them are good at this and others are not, and Patti confirms that they always know when someone other than the Solutionists has done any work on a boat: 'the standard is often very different and we

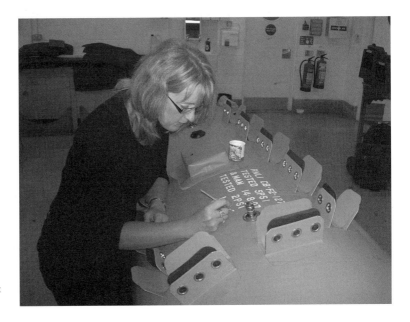

Rubber Solutionist
Sonya Wright.

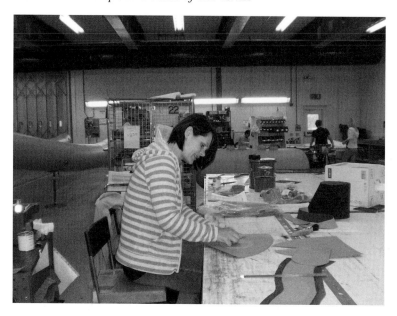

Rubber Solutionist
Belinda Masterson.

cannot risk the consequences of something failing'. Jane Atkins recalls having to re-do work to make sure that it meets the standard. Belinda Millichamp likes to put her head round the door of a boathouse to say hello when she is out and about on the coast. More than once she has been greeted with the words 'Now you're here, could you just help with this …', and she does!

With such a mighty focus on achieving the highest quality and the compelling sense of responsibility towards the crews, it is not surprising that the Solutionists feel anxious about changes in procedures and practice which they fear may jeopardise what they strive to deliver for the crews. Without question, there is immense pride in what they do, and every individual speaks with enthusiasm about when they see lifeboats on the television or at the coast. Each and every woman looks for the number of the lifeboat to see if it is one they have worked on, and each feels pride when their friends or family show an interest in what they do.

For Sue Hayward, there is 'a real sense of privilege in being a part of the RNLI and supporting the guys who go out there'. She did similar work for the MOD in Devon before moving to the Isle of Wight, but is clear that working for the RNLI is something very special. She is not daunted by the comments she hears from some members of the public with the implication that she and her colleagues '*only* build boats'. She knows such people do not understand, but she is confident in the value of what she and they do – ensuring that only the very best inshore lifeboats are provided for the crews.

The Solutionists are a unique group of people with a job that has no comparator anywhere else. What was once renowned as an all-woman department now employs men. Nicky Stokes explains that the work is, on the whole, more suited to female strengths, such as precision working, planning, multi-tasking, patience and completion. However, she and the others recognise that women do not have the monopoly of these, and male colleagues add to the team with their particular strengths.

In another part of the Inshore Lifeboat Centre is a woman who has achieved success in a predominantly male occupation. Sarah Fulford is currently a Section Leader in the Electrical Engineering team. She has come a long way from starting as a Youth Training Scheme student in 1990, but has no doubts about what motivates her at work. Sarah is always conscious that her job is to help save lives at sea. She knows that the crews depend for their safety on the equipment on their lifeboats, and therefore she and her team must ensure their work is consistently of the highest quality. She is yet another woman proud to work for the RNLI, and who is generous with praise for her team.

And finally …

Sue Hennessy, first Principal of the Lifeboat College

Two pictures in my grandparents' house made a big impression on me when I was a small girl. One was a sepia photograph of a lifeboat crew posing in front of their pulling and sailing lifeboat, and the other was a drawing of sailors climbing high up into the rigging of a sailing ship. Both had belonged to my great-grandfather, Lawrence Hennessy, who, as coxswain of Hythe lifeboat, led his crew in two rescues on 11 November 1891. As a result of their efforts and considerable courage, thirty-one lives were saved, although tragically one of his crew was killed as they launched the lifeboat into the raging surf. My great-grandfather was awarded two Silver Medals for gallantry by the RNLI and the Albert Medal, which was presented to him in person by Queen Victoria.

All his children eventually moved away from the coast and none followed their father into a lifeboat crew, but our family has always supported the RNLI. I never consciously thought about employment with the RNLI until, in 1991, I saw an advertisement for the Regional Manager in north-west England and decided to apply. It was one of the best decisions of my life! I was immediately struck by the commitment of the volunteers – on the coast and far inland. The first fundraising committee meeting I attended was at Ramsbottom, a small community in the Pennines and a long way from the sea. The energy and enterprise of the people there were outstanding, but, as I was to discover, it was the same everywhere. Many were from a generation of married women not in paid employment but using their considerable talents to benefit charitable causes. Such a contrast with my own life – I had never been to a coffee morning until I attended as an RNLI employee! Meeting such competent women presented me with much to reflect on as I could see that the loss of their contribution within the world of work was more than compensated for by the great gain for many charitable and voluntary enterprises.

For me, one of the great riches of employment with the RNLI has been the opportunity to meet and work with people with such different professional and personal backgrounds. In all parts of the organisation there are many extraordinarily competent men and women and it has been a joy to observe them and learn something that I could then put to good use. At first I was surprised to find that staff stayed with the RNLI for so long, but soon the years began to race past for me and I realised that I too had become completely immersed in the work.

Can you imagine the satisfaction of securing a major donation for the RNLI – a sum sufficient to enable the building of a new lifeboat, boathouse or other expensive project? In

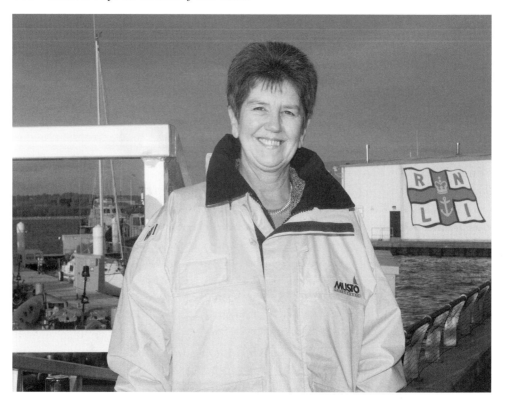

Sue Hennessy, retired College Principal/Head of Training.

my second job as Personal Donations Manager, I frequently experienced such pleasure, but it was an even greater fulfilment to discover that, for many of the donors, the experience of giving such special support brought them a whole new meaning to their life as it opened the opportunity for a personal relationship with 'their' lifeboat station. Seeing that happen many times has always made me happy.

From the moment I heard that we were to build a training college at Poole, I knew I wanted to take a leading role in developing and running it. When the advertisement appeared for the College Principal/Head of Training, I was not really hopeful of being appointed. I observed the RNLI still to be a very male dominated organisation and expected that a woman candidate had a low chance of success. My own views about female competence had been shaped by my school – a girls' school. Under the leadership of an inspiring headmistress, an early member of the Fabian Society, we were educated to regard ourselves firstly as people with unique talents and skills. People, whether girls or boys, had equal rights to develop these and to compete in the world. This philosophy has always served me well, and did so again when, following the selection process, my appointment was confirmed.

The brief was to develop the Lifeboat College as a resource for delivering high quality training for lifeboat crews, lifeguards, other volunteers and staff and to ensure it ran on a sound financial base, which would save external expenditure as well as generate income for the charity. Additionally, to create a 'home' for the RNLI to welcome all those in any way associated with its work. It was a major challenge – one that might enable me to leave a special legacy to the organisation that my great-grandfather had served so well. And so I set to work ... having first hung the picture of him and his crew taken in 1891 on my office wall. In the busy days ahead, it would give me both encouragement and inspiration.

Within these pages, there are women that I know well; women that, through writing this book, I have got to know; and yet more that I dearly wish I had known. There are even more women who, had this been an encyclopaedia, would have been included. The RNLI is alive with outstanding women working alongside equally outstanding men, ensuring that as many people as possible who find themselves in trouble, either on or by the sea, live rather than drown. It is a noble cause that unites everyone involved in the organisation.

When I first joined the RNLI as a member of staff, I was fascinated – and very impressed – by the women of such outstanding calibre and commitment that I met within the volunteer fundraising committees. Nearly twenty years later, I keep meeting more outstanding women in every part of the RNLI, and my admiration and respect for them has not yet found its limit. They are the salt of the earth.

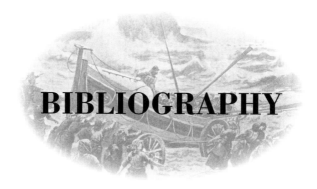

BIBLIOGRAPHY

Cox, Barry, *Lifeboat Gallantry: The Complete Record of Royal National Lifeboat Institution Gallantry Medals and How They Were Won, 1824–1996*, Savannah, 1998

Dawson, Major A. J., *Britain's Lifeboats*, Hodder and Stoughton, 1923

Kelly, Robert, *For Those in Peril*, Shearwater Press, 1979

Kilroy, F., *'The Ladies': A Century of Service*, Publisher, 1992

Kipling, R. and S., *Strong to Save*, Patrick Stephens, 1995

Kipling, R. and S., *Never Turn Back*, Sutton Publishing, 2006

Mitford, Jessica, *Grace Had an English Heart*, E.P. Dutton, 1988

Skidmore, Ian, *Lifeboat VC: The Story of Coxswain Dick Evans and His Many Rescues*, David & Charles, 1979

The Lifeboat: A Complete Historical Archive 1852–2008, RNLI Heritage Trust, 2008

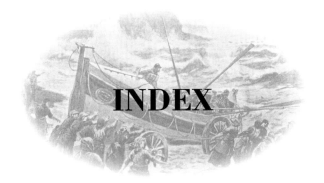

INDEX